THE ADOLESCENT
IN
GROUP AND FAMILY THERAPY

The Adolescent in Group and Family Therapy

Edited by

MAX SUGAR, M.D.

Clinical Professor of Psychiatry, Louisiana State University
School of Medicine (New Orleans)

BRUNNER/MAZEL, *Publishers*　New York

To

BARBARA, MELISSA,
DAVID, ROXANNE
AND MICHAEL

Contributors

DORIS BARTLETT, M.A.
Chief Psychologist, Gouveneur Hospital, New York City, and Assistant Clinical Professor, New York University and Teachers College, Columbia University.

IRVING H. BERKOVITZ, M.D.
Clinical Assistant Professor of Psychiatry at the University of California at Los Angeles, and a Senior Psychiatric Consultant for the Los Angeles Department of Mental Health.

DAVID A. BERKOWITZ, M.D.
Clinical Instructor at George Washington University, Washington, D. C., and Clinical Associate in Child Psychiatry, National Institute of Mental Health, Bethesda, Md.

BEATRICE M. COOPER, M.S.
Social worker on the staff of Reiss-Davis Clinic, Los Angeles.

DAVID MENDELL, M.D.
Clinical Professor of Psychiatry at the University of Texas Medical School, Houston, and Clinical Associate Professor of Psychiatry, Baylor College of Medicine, Houston.

DANIEL OFFER, M.D.
Associate Director of the Institute for Psychosomatic and Psychiatric Research and Training, Vice Chairman of the Department of Psychiatry, Michael Reese Hospital and Medical Center, and Professor of Psychiatry at the Pritzker School of Medicine, University of Chicago.

ABEL OSSORIO, Ph.D.
Regional Health Director, Public Health Service, Department of Health, Education and Welfare, Denver, Colorado.

ADOLFO E. RIZZO, M.D.
  Clinical Assistant Professor of Psychiatry, Washington University, St. Louis, Missouri.

LEONARD SAXON, M.A.
  Clinical psychologist in St. Louis, Missouri.

EDWARD R. SHAPIRO, M.D.
  Clinical Associate at the National Institute of Mental Health, Bethesda, Maryland, and member of the Department of Psychiatry and Behavioral Sciences, George Washington University, Washington, D. C.

ROGER L. SHAPIRO, M.D.
  Professor and Director of Clinical Services, Department of Psychiatry and Behavioral Sciences, George Washington University, Washington, D.C.

ROBERT A. SOLOW, M.D.
  Assistant Clinical Professor of Psychiatry, University of California at Los Angeles, and member of the staff of the Reiss-Davis Clinic, Los Angeles.

HYMAN SPOTNITZ, M.D., Med. Sc. D.
  Research psychiatrist engaged in the practice of psychoanalytic psychotherapy in New York City.

VANN SPRUIELL, M.D.
  Clinical Associate Professor of Psychiatry at Louisiana State University Medical School in New Orleans, and a Training and Supervising Analyst at the New Orleans Psychoanalytic Institute.

HELM STIERLIN, M.D., Ph.D.
  Acting Chief of the Family Studies Section of the Adult Psychiatry Branch, National Institute of Mental Health, Bethesda, Maryland, Assistant Professor of Psychiatry at the Johns Hopkins Hospital, Baltimore, Maryland, and member of the faculty of the Washington Psychoanalytic Institute, and The Washington School of Psychiatry.

MAX SUGAR, M.D.
  Clinical Professor of Psychiatry, Louisiana State University School of Medicine, New Orleans, and President of the American Society for Adolescent Psychiatry, 1973/74.

EVERT VANDERSTOEP, M.D.
> Director of the Outpatient Department of the Illinois State Psychiatric Institute in Chicago, Associate Attending Psychiatrist at Michael Reese Hospital, and Clinical Instructor in Psychiatry at the University of Illinois.

CARL A. WHITAKER, M.D.
> Professor of Psychiatry at the University of Wisconsin Merical School, Madison.

FRANK S. WILLIAMS, M.D.
> Assistant Chief of Child Psychiatry at Cedars-Sinai Medical Center in Los Angeles, Assistant Clinical Professor of Psychiatry at the University of California in Los Angeles, a faculty member of the Southern California Psychoanalytic Institute and President-Elect of the American Society for Adolescent Psychiatry, 1973/74.

JOHN ZINNER, M.D.
> Associate Professor of Psychiatry at George Washington University, Washington, D. C.

Preface

Many adolescents are unsuited for individual therapy but may be amenable to group or family therapy. Group therapy and family therapy with focus on the adolescent have come of age, with many articles and some books written on varied techniques and theories, as adjuncts or as primary methods of therapy. This does not imply that individual therapy is to be phased out; rather, at times another mode of treatment may be optimal for the designated patient. The purpose of this book is to provide a panoramic view of some of these developments in the theory and practice of group and family therapy with adolescents. Both of these modalities have extended and added immeasurably to the approaches in treating adolescents and some varieties of techniques and parameters utilized successfully by practitioners in the field are presented in this volume.

We take the view that there are many more different recipes than can possibly be included in this work, and therefore we are offering a sampling, a potpourri or a gourmet's delight, according to the reader's taste. An exhaustive encyclopedic textbook approach is eschewed in favor of the immediate experience of the authors and their application of theory to a particular patient in a particular setting.

In essence, we feel that the approaches here detailed are primarily of a psychoanalytic framework. They take cognizance of the structural theory, developmental lines, and phase-specific needs of the adolescent, such as ego, superego, ego ideal, autonomy and identity developments, and the process of separation-individuation, as well as early, middle and late adolescent concerns. Indications and contraindications are taken up in detail along with transference, resistance, and countertransference issues. Thus, we feel that a well-rounded view is offered to the practitioner involved in the decision-making process of when, why and how to use group or family therapy, with or without individual therapy.

xi

Our goal is to describe specific applications of group or family therapy to the adolescent in a variety of particular situations. Thus the writings included offer a specific focus on the adolescent in group or family therapy—his involvement with personal problems, or in community issues like a high school with problems, or with drug addiction, or in a problem family.

We hope these experiences and applications may serve as useful models for others through the application and innovation of these and other sound approaches to help adolescents with their normative, familial, environmental or intrapsychic difficulties.

ACKNOWLEDGMENTS

Grateful acknowledgments are in order for the enormous amount of encouragement and assistance given to me by many people. To name a few, I mention first, with thanks, my wife, Barbara, who provided the ambience that allowed for the effort required for this book, and invaluable kindly criticism and editorial assistance. Dr. Dan Offer encouraged me to embark on this venture and then contributed to it. Dr. Lois DeBakey gave editorial assistance. Lois Murphy patiently typed innumerable revisions with helpful comments. The Executive Committee of the American Society for Adolescent Psychiatry cheered me on.

In addition, I wish to express my appreciation to each of the authors. Thanks are extended to Basic Books for permission to reproduce "Family Therapy: Its Role in Adolescent Psychiatry" by Dr. Frank S. Williams from *Adolescent Psychiatry*, Volume 2, 1973; and the *Journal of the Academy of Child Psychiatry* for permission to reproduce my article, "Group Therapy with Pubescent Boys with Absent Fathers," from Volume 6, 1967.

Most importantly, I wish to acknowledge my debt to the many adolescents from whom I have learned so much.

MAX SUGAR, M.D.

Contents

Introduction

One of the problems those of us face who are supposed to be helpful to adolescents by means of "counseling" or "therapy" was clearly recognized by Anna Freud, way back when, and has baffled us ever since. If I may state it somewhat crudely and as briefly as possible: How do I know whether whatever they do is simply "because they are going through a developmental phase" or whether they are on the verge of going crazy, or of becoming juvenile delinquents? Or—as we know only too well, by now—maybe this special piece of atrocious behavior is really a healthy defense against the miserable conditions under which they are supposed to grow up or a rather "normal" reaction to the equally miserable things we have done to them? Or, worse even, maybe the problem behavior producer this morning falls into the "crazy" category, while similar behavior by the same kid in the afternoon belongs to the "hard to live with but basically normal" category?

In recent years a new complexity, which wasn't so clear in the early days, has become increasingly obvious—the terrific impact of "group situations" on adolescent lives. Whether we see them emigrate from their "family group" or watch them struggle with their immigration into the "peer group culture of the older or tougher kids," it is surely obvious that a new dimension has to be taken into account. So—it was only natural to wonder if forces as strong as "group ties" could also be engaged in the process of treatment, and if we could use as a therapeutic tool what first seemed as though it were primarily a force against us.

No wonder, therefore, that there has been a tendency, in the earlier publications in this field, to welcome the group as a medium with a somewhat orgiastic hope that "groups can do it better." Even people trained in the rigorous discipline of individual therapy were easily led to expect that, as soon as they would work with groups, they could ditch everything else. There has also been a trend to assume that the mere awareness of social complications and of group dynamics would guarantee beneficial therapeutic effects on a given youngster. To those who may still be tempted to hope for such an easy way out, this book should administer a wonderful "complexity shock."

The therapists who have contributed to this volume have done all their clinical and technical speculating on the basis of real, down-to-earth experiences with live youngsters—individually and in groups—in the here-and-now mess of their lives and of the larger societal turmoil of our time. What they seem to me to accomplish superbly in this volume is the following:

First, they are freeing group therapy at last from the suspicion of being ignorant of—or at least disinterested in—a depth-oriented, or even downright "Freudian," approach to the inner workings of developmental and other complications in their adolescent patients. In fact, in spite of the title of this publication and its major theme, some of the deliberations on complications and multiple meanings of such terms as "transference," "countertransference," etc. could just as well have been contained in papers restricted to the individual on the couch. This makes it even more fascinating to watch the new complications such concepts involve when applied to processes in the group.

Second, without being recklessly or smugly "eclectic," the authors of this book show a most refreshing "open mind" attitude to a wide variety of theoretical and therapeutic possibilities. Even though each remains bound to the specific theoretical slant he feels most comfortable with, they all take pains to convince the reader that whatever theoretical stance they are taking is meaningful because it fits the "here and now" of a specific situation or a specific case, with no implication that it is necessarily supposed to be "it." The healthy reminder that there are still more kids and more differences than could fit any one theoretical position runs like a refreshing breeze through this book.

And finally, this volume is also wonderfully free of some of the naiveté of some of the earlier positions often taken by group and family therapists, who so easily found themselves caught up in some form of "either-or-itis"—the most dangerous disease of our time. Indications as well as contraindications for exposing adolescents to individual, group or family treatment are discussed with admirable clinical restraint, and it is obvious that all the writers represented here are equally at home in both settings. It is a delight to see a relatively young field, such as group therapy, emerge from the unavoidable childhood diseases of any scientific movement, with no ill after effects at all.

FRITZ REDL, PH.D.
Distinguished Professor
of Behavioral Sciences (Emeritus)
Wayne State University (Detroit)

Part I
GROUP THERAPY

1

Indications and Contraindications for Adolescent Group Psychotherapy

IRVING H. BERKOVITZ, M.D.
and MAX SUGAR, M.D.

Essential to determining indications for any form of therapy for adolescents is a concept of the developmental tasks of adolescence. The concept held by the authors includes 1) emancipation from parental attachments; 2) development of satisfying and self-realizing peer attachments, with ability to love and appreciate the worth of others as well as oneself; 3) an endurable and sustaining sense of identity in the familial, social, sexual, and work-creative areas; and 4) a flexible set of hopes and life goals for the future.

In addition, while deciding need for therapy for an adolescent, one has to keep in mind that suffering in adolescents is often registered first by the immediate objects, i.e., the persons in the social system around the teenager: the family, the caretakers, the individual's social network, or the legal system. In this age group it is important to keep in mind that the boundaries between the normal and the abnormal are shifting, often fluid and frequently a matter of judgment. Of significance are the manner in which the individual copes with problems and the way the social system reacts.

If the adolescent needs treatment for other than a transient personal or situational crisis, individual therapy, group, or family therapy, or a combination of these may be considered. In some instances, the family therapy which includes several siblings offers the opportunity for periods of discussion which can resemble and provide the values of a group therapy experience within the family session. In many cases the choice

3

among these three major types of therapy is, indeed, a practical one related mostly to the circumstances of the individual teenager, his family's acceptance or finances, or the persons (individual or agency) providing the treatment. Each of these three major types of therapy provides unique advantages, benefits and complications. Frequently there is value in periods of alternation or simultaneous use of all three.

The recommendation of group therapy for the adolescent depends to a great extent on the availability of a suitable adolescent group. Unfortunately, a dearth of therapeutically oriented groups prevails in most communities. Many teenage groups, available in free clinics, schools, churches or clubs, with or without therapeutic orientation, can provide therapeutic and growth values.

In this chapter we will present some of our ideas and what many practitioners have written about the special usefulness of group therapy, with or without the concurrent presence of the other types of treatment. Indications in the inpatient as well as outpatient settings will be considered.

Small groups allow exposure of typical behavioral patterns leading to a decrease in feelings of isolation and of being peculiar, with a rise in self-esteem. Concomitantly they foster new ways of dealing with situations, along with an evaluation of techniques in use.

A prime advantage of group therapy to many teenagers is the feeling of protection vis-à-vis the adult therapist. The opportunity to rap with peers seems less associated with being ill (at first) and safer from possible adult domination. Many teenagers are curious upon first learning of group therapy as to the nature of the discussions and the possibility of making new friends. Of course, in some adolescents, especially those who fear peer relationships, an opposite reaction may prevail. The youngster's distrust of adults, beginning with parents, usually makes the peer group especially acceptable at this stage of development.

Group therapy has special value in engaging the adolescent in therapy, as noted by Peck and Bellsmith (1954), who stated:

> A properly selected group will expose the patient's characteristic distortions as they appear in the interaction between himself and certain members of the group. Since he is also capable of entering into relatively healthy relationships with certain other members of the group, he is able more easily to examine and work through his relationship distortion, because he is supported by the reassuring reality of his healthy social ties within the group.

It soon became apparent that a number of the children, who had appeared passive in individual sessions rapidly became surprisingly active in the group setting.

Buxbaum (1945) has described the violent swings from rebellion to submission that occur in adolescent groups. She felt that both processes are of equal importance for the adolescent's development since breaking away encourages independence and increases identification with the leader, while being submissive to peer approval gives him an opportunity to satisfy dependency needs in a setting where he retains control of when to terminate this role. Giving the adolescent a chance both to submit and revolt alternately is one of the characteristics, according to Buxbaum, which particularly makes the group indispensable for the adolescent. This is especially exemplified in group therapy with delinquent adolescents, detailed later in the chapter.

Group therapy may be especially indicated currently, since the "do-your-own-thing" ethos of the 1960's and '70's often encourages some teenagers to prolong a normal narcissistic orientation. Rather than learning empathy or understanding, for some teenagers manipulation or disregard of others may become more prevalent. Group therapy, experienced even briefly, may afford an opportunity to open the individual's mind to fuller appreciation of, and, hopefully, reduction of blocks to warm, honest, nonexploitative relationships with others. The group experiences available in "normal settings," that is, schools, clubs or churches, may often provide the same benefit. One has to beware, in some, however, of an emphasis on group comfort or sometimes of traumatic interpersonal encounters, instead of a slower, more gradual and tolerable pace of coming to know oneself and the other person. Josselyn (1972) cautioned of some dangers in ill-timed or too pressing a group experience.

This presentation of the values in adolescent group therapy does not signify that the group is rigidly the treatment of choice for all teenagers, with or without concurrent individual or family sessions. There are many examples of individual therapy alone in which the adolescent has developed a corrective child-adult experience that has allowed for repair of previous maturational lags and/or various symptoms. However, even in these cases, as helpful as the individual treatment may have been, a social practice arena often may have been of added value in deepening and consolidating the therapy. In many individuals (not only the very schizoid) one may encourage, suggest, and even arrange for extratherapeutic group experiences and opportunities, such as recreational clubs and other groups, but without successful involvement developing. An adolescent therapy group, on the other hand, provides this opportunity intrinsic to the therapy itself, with the excellent possibility that blocks to learning from, and sharing with, peers may be pointed out more effectively.

Group therapy, skillfully handled with attention to psychodynamic considerations, may be useful to many neurotic, antisocial, or psychotic teenagers. It may suffice as the only therapeutic experience in many mildly disturbed youngsters, but more disturbed individuals may well need the added assistance of individual and family therapy as well. The use of individual, family, or group therapy concurrently by the same therapist deserves more detailed discussion than can be given here. A communication gap may occur when two therapists are involved. However, an equally significant resistance can occur even with the single therapist when the teenager tries to avoid involvement in the individual or group relation by pitting one against the other (Brackelmanns and Berkovitz, 1972).

Relevant questions in this discussion, therefore, would be: Which teenagers are appropriate for group therapy? At which stage of individual or family therapy should group therapy be recommended? What benefit can be expected from group therapy? Or what detriment? What is the best method of recommending or preparing the individual teenager for group therapy? Which group and therapist should one choose for the particular adolescent? Some possible answers to some of these questions will be suggested in this chapter.

Some have tried, usually in the treatment of adults, to determine criteria by which to predict gain from group therapy and the most productive composition of a group (Yalom, 1970). Criteria are yet to be similarly described for adolescent group therapy. While there is rarely the ideal group, some individuals may do better in one type of group than in another, and with one particular group therapist than with another. Moreover, indications for group therapy must also include some thought about the effect of the individual on the group, since entry and premature, early termination will hurt or impede the individual, as well as the group.

The degree of indication for recommending group psychotherapy to any teenager may be crudely quantified into absolute, relative, or minimal degrees. Under absolute degree of indication, we would consider those youngsters so well defended against therapeutic relationships that only in a peer group or network group (Sugar, 1972) can there be any significant confrontation, introspection, or interaction with therapist or peers.

Minimal degree of indication would include the teenager who relates to the adult therapist fairly well. He may defy or withhold at times, but to a manageable degree, which does not prevent growth or understanding. This category of young person has meaningful group associations in some areas of his life. In many ways this adolescent's individual therapy is already proceeding beneficially, and the degree of psychological impairment may well be minimal.

The category of relative indication for group psychotherapy would be somewhere between the previous two categories. In this case, experiencing group therapy would help add greater here-and-now evidence, from interpersonal application, of changes or understanding arrived at in the one-to-one therapeutic relationship. At times, even relationship problems not previously known may be uncovered.

Once a practitioner has decided that group therapy may be useful for a teenager, the next step is to obtain agreement from the youngster for this treatment plan. If he had come requesting group therapy, as some do, there is little problem. When the teenager has been so poorly prepared for group therapy or any therapy by the parents and therapist that he denies any need for therapy, it is best not to embark on group therapy. The parental messages to him need to be examined and if the parents are mostly for the youngster being in therapy, then a preparatory period of individual therapy should be the next step. Thus he may gain some comfort with the therapist which could prepare him for the group experience. Some youngsters have such negative, suspicious feelings and expectations of getting hurt (through rejection or other painful methods) that they reject individual therapy automatically. Then group therapy may offer them an opportunity for dealing with these feelings as well as give them a possibly corrective experience.

> Members may initially come to the group under pressure; but if the group is to form and become a viable entity, members must come to feel this sense of belonging and to accept their part in the group and some responsibility for it. Thus, consent is ultimately crucial. Members come for some common purpose; but they also have their separate needs, their hidden agendas, and there will be struggles to reconcile these in the group and pressure for members to conform to the demands of the group as a whole and to reach agreement (MacLennan and Felsenfeld, 1968, p. 7).

Entry into group therapy indicates a wish by the teenager and therapist for several mutually desired changes:

(1) a greater enabling of interdependent autonomy; this would include emancipation from disabling attachments to parental demands

and expectations but allow for a respectful appreciation of and reconciliation with positive qualities of parents and other adults; (2) reduction (but not crippling) of childhood narcissism, so that there is greater ability to respond to the worth of other individuals, beginning with peers; (3) enhancing appreciation for personal creative energies, so that a sustaining life goal and zest for what is available in living become more stable features in the personality; (4) a greater sense of sureness of self, in terms of familial, sexual, and social identity, with a minimum of arrogance and rigidity (Berkovitz, 1972, p. 6).

Fried (1956) aimed at developing a "self-servicing ego" to replace the "parent servicing ego."

GROUPS IN OUTPATIENT SETTINGS

There are many types of outpatient groups. One type, conducted primarily in the office or clinic setting, emphasizes such features as mainly weekly sessions, primarily verbalized confrontation of behavior, description of feelings, interpretation and increased intellectual-emotional understanding.

Brackelmanns and Berkovitz (1972), discussing this type of group, considered as positive indications two types of resistance to forming an alliance with the therapist:

> The first of these is represented by the youngster who passively accepts his fate and allows himself to be carried back and forth to the office but refuses any involvement. There was an example of a thirteen-year-old boy who offered no overt resistance to coming to treatment but, upon arrival, sat silently for the entire time. More often than not, he appeared drowsy or fell asleep. The second form of response, more common in girls than in boys, is a more open hostile rebellion to treatment. This type of young adolescent is full of promises of failure, feelings of distrust, threats of termination, and raw insults, both personal and professional, which are directed at the therapist. . . .
>
> Two relative *contraindications* to group psychotherapy are overt psychosis and severe narcissism or nonempathy. The latter is an interesting problem which the group and therapist find difficult to deal with. This patient tends to be very verbal and preoccupied with himself and his own problems and has little genuine concern for other people. He angers the group, but they find it hard to control him because of their own narcissism, their concerns about being critical and being criticized, and the way in which this patient transmits an aura of being fragile and helpless. An attack on him (or her)

results in the attacker's feeling guilty. It has been very helpful to have this type of patient also in individual psychotherapy, and to educate him in group conduct with emphasis on developing his skills toward greater empathy and more effective interpersonal inter-action. . . .

The therapist must consider the danger of *mixing nonacting out adolescents with acting out adolescents.* It is possible that the young person, as he makes separation from his family and engages with the peer group, will identify with acting out adolescent behavior in order to gain acceptance. In addition to this process, the group often pro-vides a sanctioning body with the tendency to encourage certain kinds of acting out behavior in order to deal with feelings.

Several other contraindications need additional consideration. The young-ster who refuses, but whose refusal may be mistaken as symptomatic of anxiety (about exposure or other matters), should not come into the group unless, and until, it is clear that this anxiety has been managed suitably so that he has some positive feelings about entering the group. Sometimes, when this is not considered, the youngster may abruptly break off treat-ment, or may seemingly act out in some other way. But this may be due to the therapist not handling adequately the youngster's extreme anxiety. In one such case, the youngster, aged 13, needed his father to intervene and decide that group therapy would interfere with the son's other activi-ties. By that time the therapist had a clearer picture of the situation and he agreed to continue only with individual therapy, whereby the anxiety was managed suitably.

Another type of contraindication is illustrated in the case of a young man of 19 who requested group therapy since he had heard about it from his friend. He was not accepted for group therapy as he was impulsive, unstable, irregular in appearing for individual sessions and tangential in all his relationships, including that with the therapist. It was uncertain if he could attend the sessions regularly enough to become constructively involved. He might well have hurt the other members through disrup-tion, and not have gained anything for himself, as well.

Teicher (1966) felt from his work with groups of disturbed adolescents from economically and emotionally deprived walks of life, that the therapist could focus on:

(1) helping in the group process with the presenting problems of the youths—problems which prevented them in many instances from dealing with the psychological work of adolescence; and
(2) helping with the psychological work of adolescence, although

in many of them this could proceed if they were freed sufficiently of pathological defenses and constricting, inhibiting anxieties.

The previous authors, while recognizing the importance of individual development, would probably define as a prime indication for group therapy facilitating the development of self in *the social context*.

Many groups do not emphasize as strongly an interpretative therapeutic focus. Braverman (1966) described a fascinating use of group discussion as a *facilitative* adjunct to individual casework therapy in an outpatient clinic. The lounge was open two nights per week for three hours each night, and the adolescents who had individual interviews on those nights were invited to drop in before or after individual sessions. A casual light atmosphere was encouraged, so they could just sit around and talk, or play games. This group was felt to help alleviate anxieties at the outset of treatment, and provide support in coping with varied everyday problems such as homework, parental controls, relationships with the opposite sex or spending money. She felt that the group provided "useful, humane ego support" to allow for sustained individual treatment. This may have been confirmed by the finding that only one teenager left individual treatment.

A very different group of adolescents, aged 13 to 15, most of whose parents were on welfare, were at times given carfare, excuses from school, food, play equipment, and occasional trips (Stranahan, et al., 1957). After this treatment of their deprivation, the boys were able to identify with the therapists, function better in school and in the community, and want individual therapy. Stebbins (1972) responded to a need and met with a group of black teenagers in a housing project. She arrived at the following helpful insights:

> 1. Adolescents who are completely unaware of the process known as "therapy" can learn the "patient" role as easily as many other people involved in psychotherapy. For those youngsters whose emotional problems are compounded by reality problems, it is better to curtail this. It is not advisable to encourage ventilation and insight production as the sole purpose for group activity. It is more rewarding for both adolescent and therapist to place primary emphasis on action *resulting* from an intrapsychic focus. There can also be some experiential, recreational, social, and informational values to groups for teenagers.
>
> 2. Not always, but many times, in a minority community, the peer group or the neighborhood group is a stronger group than the family group. This peer group then becomes a more natural group with which to work. In this way, the individual appears to be more able

to satisfy his needs and build the skills he lacks. The transition of these skills to other groups and to nongroup life situations appears to be facilitated by working with whatever group is natural.

3. Privacy and closure are especially important in working with youths whose day-to-day lives bring them in constant contact with each other. For psychotherapy to have any value or to be respected at all as a helping process, it must allow for this privacy.

4. A therapist offering help to a group of oppressed adolescents must have more to offer than his clinical skills. Commonality of background, life-style, or mode of communication helps greatly. As one human being who has some realistic perception of the pitfalls encountered by other human beings, you must offer something for these young men and women to hold onto. You must extend yourself, your time, and your mind. This increases greatly your chances of receiving reciprocal sincerity (Stebbins, 1972).

MacLennan (1967) has long been an ardent advocate of the values of this type of group conducted in the indigenous setting. Sugar (see Chapter 8) used a somewhat related approach in dealing with a high school crisis.

DELINQUENT ADOLESCENTS IN OUTPATIENT GROUPS

In other outpatient settings, the teenagers are more severely delinquent, angry and uncooperative. Again, approaches can vary between the more therapeutically oriented interpretive mode therapy group to the more indigenous discussion style activity group. In the situation of delinquent youth, indications and contraindications for group techniques vary with the type of delinquent being served. Redl (1966) described four types of delinquency usually encountered: (1) delinquency as a defense in basically healthy individuals; (2) delinquency in adolescent acute growth confusional states; (3) delinquencies on a neurotic basis; and (4) delinquency based on deformities of the psychical system. Indications and style of group can vary further, depending on whether the setting is outpatient, institutional, or residential.

In an outpatient group of delinquent boys, aged 14 to 17, Jacobs and Christ (1967) developed three guiding principles for treatment of this type of group:

(1) providing outlets for tension reduction,

(2) formal structuring, and

(3) flexible setting of limits.

In two groups of delinquent adolescents, the fortuitous availability of the group as a forum helped avoid imminent physical combat in the streets (Rachman, 1969; O'Shea, 1972).

Furthermore, group therapy has been seen to deepen and maintain the involvement of these action-oriented youngsters in examination of action and feeling (Peck and Bellsmith, 1954). Their follow-up indicated that "Of all the adolescents placed in groups after failure in individual therapy, about 60 percent achieved varying degrees of improvement."

While most groups meet weekly, some therapists make a special point of the need to meet more often (Franklin and Nottage, 1969). These authors reported that by treating

> seriously disturbed delinquents in psychoanalytic group therapy five times a week, where direct focus on personality exploration is explicit and consistently maintained from the outset, it is possible to involve them successfully in deeply meaningful and highly productive understanding of themselves.

They claimed that adolescents considered untreatable by others were helped in this type of group experience.

Heacock (1966) urged that

> . . . in our experience, the most important tool the therapist has is the strong positive transference. The therapist must have a tolerance for lateness and absences but must apply consistently firm pressure to get the patient to change this behavior. He must work generally in the framework of a very positive transference constantly reaching out by phone, mail, telegrams, or home visits.

He listed as not suited for his type of group therapy

> the acting-out boy whose antisocial behavior is not nearly as severe as that of the other boys. He is made too anxious by the discussions and behavior of the rest of the group.

> Another unsuitable type is the severely delinquent and hyperactive boy who "acts in" during the sessions. His disruptive behavior spreads to the others who are quite responsive to this, and so therapy becomes impossible. Suggestible patients who are easily led should be eliminated, as they are frequently stimulated to more acting out by the therapy. Often these are borderline mental defectives. Boys presenting overt homosexual behavior are also unsuitable.

Positive reinforcement techniques, along with group discussion, are used by some. Pascal, Cottrell, and Baugh (1967) recounted the use of videotapes with five boys, aged 12 to 18, who were referred from juvenile court, charged with offenses from petty larceny to attempted murder.

James, et al., (1967) conducted a reinforcement type of "self-concept" group for 14 girls aged 13 to 17. These girls had been "runaways, court cases, and school dropouts. Three were potentially suicidal, rebellious, and acting out sexually." The group's focus was

> on charm and grooming, while selected female leaders provided role models. Discussion was like group therapy. Draw-a-person tests and check lists showed changes suggesting greater feminine identification, less hostility to authority, and greater openness to criticism after 12 weeks.

The authors felt "it was not threatening, as group therapy might have been, but the group leader was able to carry discussion into areas that would have been considered in group therapy."

INDICATIONS AND CONTRAINDICATIONS FOR ADOLESCENT GROUP THERAPY IN HOSPITALS

A necessary question, when one considers this setting, is the indication or contraindication of the previously detailed types of small groups with adolescents alongside the variety of group experiences offered in a therapeutic hospital milieu. In some large public hospitals with less abundant therapeutic facilities, the small group may have a more special therapeutic indication (Powdermaker and Frank, 1953).

Rinsley (1972) made several important points of the pertinence of the small group experience in the hospital milieu.

> A . . . consideration has to do with the timing of the prescription for the adolescent inpatient's inclusion in a therapeutic group, which is closely linked to whether the adolescent is yet immersed in the "resistance phase" of his treatment, or has passed beyond it, made therapeutic identifications with the ward or cottage staff members, hence has begun to perceive the residential setting as potentially helpful to him.
>
> In numerous cases, initiation of formal group psychotherapy while the adolescent continues actively or covertly to resist the therapeutic milieu as a whole simply intensifies the resistances, spreads them out, as it were, and abets the adolescent's use of splitting defenses, now carried over, in addition, to the "group." By the same token, attentively conducted and properly structured groups which meet directly in the patients' living areas serve to minimize the clinical-administra-

tive splits which adolescents so readily exploit from fear of self-revelation, hence may actually supply motivation for treatment.

A . . . matter concerns the use of group psychotherapy in the residential setting in conjunction with ongoing individual psychotherapy. Despite his artful and often stentorian resistances against "closeness," the adolescent inpatient, like his otherwise healthy brother in the community, struggles mightily with the problems and attainment of intimacy. As he works on object removal and proceeds to devalue parents and their transference equivalents from anxiety over the prospect of regressive re-fusion with them, he nonetheless assiduously pursues closeness as prefatory to the capacity for later, mature object relations. In part for these reasons, group treatment without concomitant or parallel individual treatment proves inadequate for the adolescent inpatient, both as an opportunity for working through problems with object removal and as a means of exploring and resolving highly delicate, personal issues which are exceedingly difficult if not impossible to express within the peer group.

Blaustein and Wolff (1972) found that after three months of conducting a small group of teenagers on a mixed (adolescent and adult) ward in a large general hospital,

> There was a distinct decrease in friction between adolescents and staff and adolescents and adult patients. From the experience with our adolescent group thus far, we are impressed by this form of treatment as a way of reaching teenagers. The stresses experienced by the adolescent patient in the intimacy of a one-to-one relationship seem to diminish within the group. Intensity is diffused, demands on the individual patient are fewer, and therefore, there is less need to defy for the sake of defiance. The result seems to be that dependency needs may be revealed and dealt with in a growth-producing way. There is the possibility of learning to talk intimately without use of drugs as a crutch, admitting to enjoyment of the spotlight, along with learning to share it, and talking openly with authority figures in a mutually respectful way.

In another small hospital, an adolescent group served therapeutically, but also as an administrative program development unit (Grold, 1972). Group discussions included discipline and suggestions for change in program, e.g., the buying of an old car for teenage boys to work on, setting up cooking and sewing for the girls, setting up dances, etc. There was a "dramatic lessening of destructive behavior. Testing of the limits of the staff advisors continued, but to a considerably lessened degree."

Moadel (1970) gave an account of successful use of a group therapy program on a female adolescent ward.

Group discussions are seen to have a value in an occupational therapy activities program as well (Mack and Barnum, 1966). ". . . the group meetings deepened greatly the meaning and therapeutic impact of the hospital experience" and resulted "in the development of close object ties with the leader and one another, in greater cohesion on the ward."

INDICATIONS FOR ADOLESCENT GROUP PSYCHOTHERAPY
IN RESIDENTIAL SETTINGS

In residential settings designed usually for delinquent teenagers or those with family problems which require placement, still other uses of group therapy have been depicted. Again, the question regarding the therapeutic contribution of small-group psychotherapy alongside other treatment modalities in the setting must be considered. Redl (Redl and Wineman, 1957; Redl, 1966) has written extensively on this approach.

In a series of three articles, Persons and associates (Persons, 1966 and 1967; Persons and Pepinsky, 1966) highlighted the therapeutic values of group therapy with individual psychotherapy in reducing recidivism of incarcerated delinquents. The occurrence of negative transference in group is associated with positive therapeutic benefit by Truax (1971), who felt that "It may be that the occurrence of negative feelings towards the therapist as an authority figure leads to some resolution" of difficulty in relating to authority figures.

Evans (1966), carrying on "analytic group therapy at government-approved schools" in England, concluded that in the group setting

> . . . Most of the delinquents are increasingly able to look at difficulties, tolerate anxiety, and not run away from their problems. They have been able to modify their aggressive outbursts and use their aggression more constructively.

A therapy group in a probation department girls' residential treatment center underwent dramatic changes when the group, having previously met in the therapists' office, assembled instead in the girls' living unit (Pottharst and Gabriel, 1972). Rinsley (1972) stressed this point also.

The fact that the previous groups met five times per week undoubtedly added to a more significant therapeutic impact. Elias (1968) depicted a five-days-per-week program in a residential setting for delinquent boys (Highfields) termed "guided group interaction." Attendance was not compulsory. The group leader often played "a relatively active part." The total program and type of delinquent boys undoubtedly were critical factors, in addition to the groups, but "after one year of freedom in the community only 16.5 percent of the Highfields boys, as compared with 48.9 percent of the boys from the state reformatory, engaged in new delinquencies."

In contrast to this frequency, Wolk and Reid (1964) claimed to demonstrate "that changes can and do occur when inmates in detention are offered group psychotherapy for only eight weeks," meeting twice per week for 1½ hours, a total of 16 sessions.

Fortunately, some authors attempted more structured evaluation of group psychotherapy in the residential setting. Taylor (1967), in a girls' borstal in New Zealand, conducted a rigorous experiment

> . . . using (1) three comparable control groups of 11 borstal girls, (2) an experimental variable of group psychotherapy over 40 weekly sessions of one and three-quarters hour each, (3) an adequate range of pretherapy and posttherapy measures, including introspective reports, rating scales, objective, reliable, and valid personality tests, and social action effects, and (4) a follow-up period.
>
> The results established that the borstal girls demonstrated improvement in the absence of treatment, more improvement with the moderate treatment of group counseling, and most improvement from group psychotherapy. The differential rate of improvement in the three groups indicates that neither a placebo effect nor spontaneous remission was an important factor in the results.
>
> At the end of the experiment, the Experimental Group members were less radical, less criminal in attitudes and behavior, and more outgoing, reflective, and interdependent. They expressed guilt for their behavior and had positive attitudes toward the borstal and probation officers. The Experimental Group was, in fact, released before the other two groups, but the difference was not statistically significant.

In residential settings with a less delinquent population, other changes were noted. In one such setting, adolescent and preadolescent boys with "learning difficulties concomitant with emotional disturbances," when involved in small groups (six or seven members), "improved their interpersonal relationships to a greater degree than did those in individual therapy, particularly their work-oriented relationships" (Mordock, et al., 1969).

In a voluntary child placement agency, groups were useful for maturing sexual attitudes (Berkovitz, et al., 1966). Group therapy was initiated originally as a way of increasing therapeutic contact with children who had not been successfully reached in previous individual casework relationships.

Pregnant Teenagers

Adolescent pregnancy, especially among the unwed, will involve characterologic factors, as well as important identity issues. Therefore, group experience with these girls often needs to extend beyond the period of pregnancy alone. One group for girls aged 13 to 16 continued for a year and a half, though all the girls had delivered after four months of group therapy.

> A combination of group therapy and group counseling, orientation, and education was used, not only with the patient, but with her mother as well. The goal with the parent was educative, geared toward helping resolve antagonisms and hostilities in the family of the patient. Group treatment with the girls demonstrated the need of oral gratification for these emotionally deprived patients (Kaufmann and Deutsch, 1967).

Barclay (1969) did not involve parents but narrated a two-year group experience in which "the sense of frustration and hopelessness appreciably diminished as mutual support developed in the group meetings and outside." After the two years, all except two (of the nine) were involved in work, training, or continuing education.

Even in obstetrical clinics, primigravid adolescents respond better to health education programs when in peer groups, after they feel like part of the group (Barnard, 1970). Visits made to members who had delivered their babies, and to the delivery room, helped further to reduce fear about impending delivery.

Drug-Abusing Adolescents

Use and abuse of marijuana, barbiturates, psychedelics, psychoactive drugs, and heroin may occasion entry into treatment before or after legal intervention. Methadone projects often include group discussion. In office, school or clinic groups many of these youngsters have found some new understanding of self, leading to a change in patterns of chemical usage, as well as occasional personality change.

In more severe cases, group therapy, with or without individual or family therapy, may not appreciably alter the self-destructive use of these substances (see Bartlett, Chapter 17 of this volume). A more totally involving community structure which can bring about self-knowledge and new life-styles is necessary. Youngsters involved in moderate drug use who live in stable, caring families may at times find benefit in the outpatient group, individual, or family approaches previously described (Brackelmanns and Berkovitz, 1972). Slagle and Silver (1972) pointed out the value of an involving group experience for depressed drug users in a clinic.

To meet the needs of the more disturbed youngsters, many communal living arrangements have been established. Many of these include intense, small group interactions (Casriel, 1963; Shelly and Bassin, 1965; Levitt, 1968) which differ in each setting. At Daytop Village one of the principal methods for "achieving self-image and behavioral change" is three-time-a-week group encounter therapy.

> Many professionals are abashed and frightened by the fierceness of the attack therapy. But Dr. Lewis Yablonsky, research consultant to Synanon, after his first 25 sessions, found that the group "attack" was an act of love in which was entwined the assumption: "If we did not care about you or have concern for you, we would not bother to point out something that might reduce your psychic pain or clarify something for you that might save your life" (Bassin, 1968).

When communal settings are not available, hospital settings are used. Here the small therapy group has particular usefulness. As some "addicts" expressed it:

> "Alone in hospital you forget what you are in for, but in an addicts' group other addicts don't allow you to forget!"
> It was felt that "mixed" arrangements would help particularly in preventing girls from becoming too difficult with each other, and such groups should have a preponderance of boys . . . the majority prefer a heterogeneous mixing with non-drug-dependent patients, and with very rare exceptions dislike mixing with other "mental" patients, preferring alcoholics despite all their grievances against them. . . . "Addicts must learn there are other people in the world, with similar problems, who are able to overcome them, people who are experienced and mature and who work." Living with non-addicts "brings you down to earth, helps you cope with problems, teaches you tolerance . . . you didn't realize before how irresponsible you were" (Glatt, 1967).

However, the results are not clearly positive in all approaches for the problems of youngsters who abuse drugs, as Bartlett describes in Chapter 17.

Obese Adolescents

The literature describing group therapy for obese adolescents is meager. With this oral control problem, just as with drug abuse and alcoholism, group methods need to include a wider social context. With obesity this may be residential camp, weight-reducing programs, or hospitals.

In one program, eleven adolescents were hospitalized in a children's chronic disease hospital for six weeks and then followed for a year.

> The inpatient phase consisted of an intensive program including group and individual therapy, recreation, exercise, dietary education, etc. During the outpatient phase, the groups were seen at monthly intervals. The parents were involved during the entire program.
> At the end of the program, three patients were still below their admission weight, three were holding their weights steady, and the remaining five had gained weight (Stanley et al., 1968).

On the other hand, when the treatment program is less aggressive, the group may be useful as an adjunct to the program. In an adolescent medical clinic, it was reported that

> While group work . . . appeared to produce an improvement in appearance and in the attitudes toward obesity, we could not show it to be any more effective than individual treatment in achieving long-term weight loss. Group therapy did provide an opportunity for socialization and for handling other conflicts (Hammar, et al., 1971).

Adolescents in Foster Homes and Welfare Programs

Children in foster homes have usually undergone a loss of family, deliberately or inadvertently. Engagement with other children in the foster home or with foster parents may be blocked by conscious or unconscious hostility, depression and other factors.

> The climate of the group, which lends itself to the development of self-confidence in the adolescent and trust in the leader, has definite carryover into life. Through the groups, many adolescent foster children are now able to handle some of their unresolved feelings concerning their natural parents and, as a result, have better relations with their foster parents (Carter, 1968).

Outpatient groups have proved useful in one department of public welfare in *avoiding placement in a foster home*. Eight non-delinquent teenagers attended weekly for one hour, in two groups, one for those under 15 and one for those older.

> They have served as an alternative to placement. The sessions provide a means of diagnosing the quality of an adolescent's peer and authority relationships as well as other aspects of his functioning.
>   These meetings have accomplished what they set out to do: provide an ego-building experience and help the members move on to other constructive social outlets (Riegel, 1968).

Adolescent Retardates

The degree of impairment of teenage retardates is of significant importance, as much or more so as in group procedures with neurotic, delinquent, or other adolescents.

> One . . . finds reports of groups composed of individuals who have nothing in common other than the fact that they have been subsumed under a societal role definition, "retarded." . . . There have been situations in which delinquent retardates, culturally deprived retardates, mongoloids, brain-damaged youngsters, and so on have constituted a poorly composed group (Borenzweig, 1970).

Participation in a group work program has been reported as increasing the verbal capacities of moderately and mildly retarded adolescents (Rafel and Stockhammer, 1961). With mildly retarded, hyperactive, behaviorally disturbed adolescent and young adult girls, group therapy helped 37 of 56 to move from being inmates on a closed ward "to learning a repertoire of behaviors that facilitated their return to community living" (Fine and Dawson, 1964).

Most of the group therapy or group work described in the literature occurred in workshops or institutions. Some outpatient groups have been reported in conjunction with school classes for the educable mentally retarded. As in the case of the psychotic, delinquent, obese, or drugabusing teenager, the retardate also often has to be treated in a therapeutic community setting, which involves training and socialization, as well as small group therapy. Consequently, the same issues arise, namely, the role of small group therapy in the wider therapeutic context.

In workshops for mildly retarded adolescents (IQ 50-70), Bellis and Sklar (1969) felt that the "group experience of the shop is a stress situation in itself." In one workshop, "mildly and moderately retarded trainees made excellent use of group process . . ." (Rosen and Rosen, 1969). The small group provided (1) a reference point for change in the lives of the trainees, allowing support of peers to help in renouncing previous "dys-functional patterns of behavior"; (2) a forum for reality testing; (3) a place to receive encouragement from peers; as well as (4) facilitation of a new set of values and attitudes compatible with the wider society. They found role playing especially useful in this regard. After six months they observed that "the therapist no longer played an active role," and con-cerns raised moved into the area of interpersonal relationships. The more retarded members of the group became more participatory and verbal.

In institutions, more disturbed and lower IQ retardates may be in-volved. In this setting, Sternlicht (1966) decided, "Activity and other nonverbal techniques are the method of choice in the group psycho-therapeutic treatment of delinquent adolescent retardates." Miezio (1967), in working with groups of perhaps less delinquent retardates, affirmed gains similar to those described for nonretarded adolescents. Groups were able to

> enhance social awareness, elevate self-concept, diminish egocentricity, improve impulse control, externalize aggression, and develop ap-propriate sublimations. Sexual identity problems were explored and clarified. Separation from home and family, the dominant theme in all of their lives, was, to some extent, worked through and accepted.

In another institution, after 67 sessions over eight months,

> the utilization of moderately structured directive group counseling methods helped to realize the goals of the project: the reduction of acting out behavior, the increase of educational and/or work placement functioning to a higher level, and the further integration and acceptance by the patients of their assets within their own life situation (Rotman and Golburgh, 1967).

Psychodrama was used by Pankratz and Buchan (1966) in treating retarded delinquents in a hospital setting and they concluded, "The director should be manipulative and directive." Begab (1962) raised a critical note in general about the use of group work with retardates:

> Actually, some of the "group" programs currently in effect are lacking many of the elements inherent in the group process. There is little, if any, interaction between the members and a common purpose or problem does not emerge. The members look to the group leader

rather than to each other for the fulfillment of certain needs. In the absence of this necessary interdependence, communication is slow to develop and the individual's role in the group is poorly defined. When these conditions prevail and group dynamics are relatively inoperative, the true value of the group experience is lost. Group sanctions do not emerge, social controls are minimized, and there is little impact on the behavior, attitudes, and values of members.

Rather than constituting a rejection of the indication of group methods for these teenagers, the criticism offered by Begab seems to underline the need for a special directive, leader-oriented element in groups of retardates. Bigman (1961) stated that the worker must be the central person, because severely retarded young adults do not have the social or task skills necessary for interdependent participation with other members of the group. Borenzweig (1970) also confirmed that "even those groups of retardates that appeared to have little structure, interdependence between members, impact on the individual retardate, or concern with problems external to the group" had the power to exert a beneficial effect upon the retardate. The individuals were changing without significant change in group structures in the process.

SUMMARY

The variety and array of different formats and settings within which groups of adolescents gather or are brought together for new understanding are indeed impressive! A few simple generalities to describe the themes and indications are certainly inadequate.

Some of the indications for groups for adolescents can be listed as follows:

> to support assistance and confrontation from peers;
> to provide a miniature real life situation for study and change of behavior;
> to stimulate new ways of dealing with situations and developing new skills of human relations;
> to stimulate new concepts of self and new models of identification;
> to feel less isolated;
> to provide a feeling of protection from the adult while undergoing changes;
> as a bind to therapy to help maintain continued self-examination;
> to allow the swings of rebellion or submission which will encourage independence and identification with the leader;
> to uncover relationship problems not evident in individual therapy.

In some settings, indications may include the above or may include also special indications related to the needs of the particular population being served or particular setting, for example, hospitals, residential centers, or detention centers for delinquent teenagers.

Contraindications are few and involve primarily the exclusion of an adolescent who is too deviant from the rest of the particular group. This is determined by the therapeutic needs of the individual, the goals and the availability of a suitable group where the youngster is not an isolate. This is not a precisely determinable relationship and often is a matter of judgment, or trial and error. Some teenagers categorized as "narcissistic" may require individual therapy to help them make a successful relation in a group, if that proves possible. Youngsters with deficient controls may benefit from individual and family therapy as outpatients, but group therapy may be inadvisable due to potential excess group contagion or stimulation leading to disorganization.

REFERENCES

BARCLAY, L. E. (1969). A group approach to young unwed mothers. *Social Casework*, 50:379-384.

BARNARD, J. E. (1970). Peer group instruction for primigravid adolescents. *Nursing Outlook*, Vol. 18, No. 8, pp. 42-43.

BASSIN, A. (1968). Daytop Village. *Psychology Today*, 2 (7):48-52.

BEGAB, M. J. (1962). Recent Developments in Mental Retardation and their Implications for Social Group Work. In *Proceedings, Institute, Social Group Work with the Mentally Retarded: Program as a Tool*. M. Schreiber, ed., pp. 1-12. New York: Association for the Help of Retarded Children.

BELLIS, J. M., and SKLAR, N. E. (1969). The challenge: Adjustment of retarded adolescents in a workshop. *Journal of Rehabilitation*, 35:19-21.

BERKOVITZ, I. H., CHIKAHISA, P., LEE, M. L., and MURASAKI, E. M. (1966). Psychosexual development of latency-age children and adolescents in group therapy in a residential setting. *International Journal of Group Psychotherapy*, 16:344-356.

BERKOVITZ, I. H. (1972). On Growing a Group: Some Thoughts on Structure, Process, and Setting. In *Adolescents Grow in Groups*, I. H. Berkovitz, ed. pp. 6-28, New York: Brunner/Mazel.

BIGMAN, E. (1961). Group Work with a Group of Severely Retarded Young Adults. In *Proceedings, Institute, Social Group Work with the Mentally Retarded*. M. Schreiber, ed., pp. 32-37. New York: Association for the Help of Retarded Children.

BLAUSTEIN, F., and WOLFF, H. (1972). Adolescent Group: A "Must" on a Psychiatric Unit—Problems and Results. In *Adolescents Grow in Groups*, I. H. Berkovitz, ed., pp. 181-191. New York: Brunner/Mazel.

BORENZWEIG, H. (1970). Social group work in the field of mental retardation: A review of the literature. *Social Science Review*, 44:177-183.

BRACKELMANNS, W. E., and BERKOVITZ, I. H. (1972). Younger Adolescents in Group Psychotherapy: A Reparative Superego Experience. In *Adolescents Grow in Groups*. I. H. Berkowitz, ed., pp. 37-48. New York: Brunner/Mazel.

BRAVERMAN, S. (1966). The informal peer group as an adjunct to treatment of the adolescent. *Social Casework*, 47:152-157.

BUXBAUM, E. (1945). Transference and group formation in children and adolescents. *Psychoanalytic Study of the Child,* 1:351-365.

CARTER, W. W. (1968). Group counseling for adolescent foster children. *Children,* 15:22-27.

CASRIEL, D. (1963). *So Fair a House: Story of Synanon.* Englewood, New Jersey: Prentice Hall, Inc.

ELIAS, A. (1968). Group treatment program for juvenile delinquents. *Child Welfare,* 47:281-290.

EVANS, J. (1966). Analytic group therapy with delinquents. *Adolescence,* 1:180-196.

FINE, R., and DAWSON, J. C. (1964). A therapy program for the mildly retarded adolescent. *American Journal of Mental Deficiency,* 69:23-30.

FRANKLIN, G., and NOTTAGE, W. (1969). Psychoanalytic treatment of severely disturbed juvenile delinquents in a therapy group. *International Journal of Psychotherapy.* 19:165-175.

FRIED, E. (1956). Ego emancipation through group psychotherapy. *International Journal of Group Psychotherapy.* 5:358-373.

GLATT, M. M. (1967). Group therapy with young drug addicts—The addicts' point of view. *Nursing Times,* 63:519-521.

GROLD, L. J. (1972). The Value of a "Youth Group" to Hospitalized Adolescents. In *Adolescents Grow in Groups.* I. H. Berkovitz, ed., pp. 192-196. New York: Brunner/Mazel.

HAMMAR, S. L., CAMPBELL, V., and WOOLLEY, J. (1971). Treating adolescent obesity. *Clinical Pediatrics,* 10:46-52.

HEACOCK, D. R. (1966). Modifications of the standard techniques for out-patient group psychotherapy with delinquent boys. *Journal of National Medical Association,* 58:41-47.

JACOBS, M. A., and CHRIST, J. (1967). Structuring and limit setting as techniques in the group treatment of adolescent delinquents. *Community Mental Health Journal,* 3:237-244.

JAMES, S. L., OSBORN, F., and OETTING, E. R. (1967). Treatment for delinquent girls: The adolescent self-concept group. *Community Mental Health Journal,* 3:377-381.

JOSSELYN, I. M. (1972). Adolescent Group Therapy: Why, When, and a Caution. In *Adolescents Grow in Groups,* I. H. Berkovitz, ed., pp. 1-5. New York: Brunner/Mazel.

KAUFMANN, P. N., and DEUTSCH, A. L. (1967). Group therapy for pregnant unwed adolescents in the prenatal clinic of a general hospital. *International Journal of Group Psychotherapy,* 17:309-320.

LEVITT, L. (1968). Rehabilitation of narcotics addicts among lower-class teenagers. *American Journal of Orthopsychiatry,* 38:56-62.

MACK, J. E., and BARNUM, M. C. (1966). Group activity and group discussion in the treatment of hospitalized psychiatric patients. *International Journal of Group Psychotherapy,* 16:452-462.

MACLENNAN, B. W. (1967). The group as reinforcer of reality: A positive approach in the treatment of adolescents. *American Journal of Orthopsychiatry,* (Digest Issue), 37:272-273.

MACLENNAN, B. W. and FELSENFELD, N. (1968). *Group Counseling and Psychotherapy with Adolescents.* New York: Columbia University Press.

MIEZIO, S. (1967). Group therapy with mentally retarded adolescents in institutional settings. *International Journal of Group Psychotherapy,* 17:321-327.

MOADEL, Y. (1970). Adolescent group psychotherapy in a hospital setting. *American Journal of Psychoanalysis,* 30:68-72.

MORDOCK, J. B., ELLIS, M. H., and GREENSTONE, J. L. (1969). The effects of group and individual therapy on sociometric choice of disturbed institutionalized adolescents. *International Journal of Group Psychotherapy,* 19:510-517.

O'SHEA, C. (1972). "Two Gray Cats Learn How It Is" in a Group of Black Teenagers. In *Adolescents Grow in Groups.* I. H. Berkovitz, ed., pp. 134-148. New York: Brunner/Mazel.

PANKRATZ, L. D., and BUCHAN, L. G. (1966). Techniques of the warm-up in psychodrama with the retarded. *Mental Retardation,* 4:12-15.

PASCAL, G. R., COTTRELL, T. B., and BAUGH, J. R. (1967). A methodological note in the use of videotape in group psychotherapy with juvenile delinquents. *International Journal of Group Psychotherapy,* 17:248-251.

PECK, H. B., and BELLSMITH, V. (1954). *Treatment of the Delinquent Adolescent.* New York: Family Service Association of America.

PERSONS, R. W. (1966). Psychological and behavioral change in delinquents following psychotherapy. *Journal of Clinical Psychology,* 22:337-340.

PERSONS, R. W. (1967). Relationship between psychotherapy with institutionalized boys and subsequent community adjustment. *Journal of Consulting Psychology,* 31:137-141.

PERSONS, R. W. and PEPINSKY, H. B. (1966). Convergence in psychotherapy with delinquent boys. *Journal of Counseling Psychology,* 13:329-334.

POTTHARST, K. E., and GABRIEL, M. (1972). The Peer Group as a Treatment Tool in a Probation Department Girls' Residential Treatment Center. In *Adolescents Grow in Groups,* I. H. Berkovitz, ed., pp. 225-232. New York: Brunner/Mazel.

POWDERMAKER, F. B., and FRANK, J. D. (1953). *Group Psychotherapy: Studies in Methodology of Research and Therapy.* Cambridge: Harvard University Press.

RACHMAN, A. W. (1969). Talking it out rather than fighting it out: Prevention of a delinquent gang war by group therapy intervention. *International Journal of Group Psychotherapy,* 19:518-521.

RAFEL, S., and STOCKHAMMER, R. (1961). The impact of a community group work agency in serving a retardate and his family. In *Proceedings, Institute, Social Group Work with the Mentally Retarded.* M. Schreiber, ed. New York: Association for the Help of Retarded Children.

REDL, F., and WINEMAN, D. (1957). *The Aggressive Child.* Glencoe, Illinois: The Free Press.

REDL, F. (1966). *When We Deal with Children.* New York: The Free Press.

RIEGEL, B. (1968). Group meetings with adolescents in child welfare. *Child Welfare,* 47:417-427.

RINSLEY, D. B. (1972). Group Therapy within the Wider Residential Context. In *Adolescents Grow in Groups.* I. H. Berkovitz, ed., pp. 233-242. New York: Brunner/Mazel.

ROSEN, H. G., and ROSEN, S. (1969). Group therapy as an instrument to develop a concept of self-worth in the adolescent and young adult mentally retarded. *Mental Retardation,* 7:52-55.

ROTMAN, C. B., and GOLBURGH, S. J. (1967). Group counseling mentally retarded adolescents. *Mental Retardation,* 5:13-16.

SHELLY, J. A., and BASSIN, A. (1965). Daytop Lodge—a new treatment approach for drug addicts. *Corrective Psychiatry and Journal of Social Therapy,* 11:186-195.

SLAGLE, P. A. and SILVER, D. S. (1972). "Turning On" the Turned Off: Active Techniques with Depressed Drug Users in a County Free Clinic. In *Adolescents Grow in Groups,* I. H. Berkovitz, ed., pp. 108-121. New York: Brunner/Mazel.

STANLEY, E. J., GLASER, H. H., LEVIN, D. G., ADAMS, P. A., and COLEY, I. L. (1968). The treatment of adolescent obesity: Is it worthwhile? *American Journal of Orthopsychiatry,* Digest issue, 38, 207.

STEBBINS, D. B. (1972). "Playing It by Ear," in Answering the Needs of a Group of

Black Teen-Agers. In *Adolescents Grow in Groups*. I. H. Berkovitz, ed., pp. 126-133. New York: Brunner/Mazel.

STERNLICHT, M. (1966). Treatment approaches to delinquent retardates. *International Journal of Group Psychotherapy*. 16:91-93.

STRANAHAN, M., SCHWARTZMAN, C., and ATKIN, E. (1957). Group treatment for emotionally disturbed and potentially delinquent boys and girls. *American Journal of Orthopsychiatry*, 27:518-527.

SUGAR, M. (1972). Psychotherapy with the Adolescent in Self-Selected Peer Groups. In *Adolescents Grow in Groups*. I. H. Berkovitz, ed., pp. 80-94. New York: Brunner/Mazel.

TAYLOR, A. J. (1967). An evaluation of group psychotherapy in a girls' borstal. *International Journal of Group Psychotherapy*, 17:168-177.

TEICHER, J. D. (1966). Group psychotherapy with adolescents. *California Medicine*, 105:18-21.

TRUAX, C. B. (1971). Degree of negative transference occurring in group psychotherapy and client outcome in juvenile delinquents. *Journal of Clinical Psychology*, 21:132-136.

WOLK, R. L., and REID, R. (1964). A study of group psychotherapy results with youthful offenders in detention. *Group Psychotherapy and Psychodrama*, 17:56-60.

YALOM, I. D. (1970). *The Theory and Practice of Group Psychotherapy*. New York: Basic Books.

2

Adolescent Narcissism and Group Psychotherapy

Vann Spruiell, M.D.

INTRODUCTION

Young adolescents are particularly "narcissistic," as everyone knows. That is, they love themselves, or attempt to love themselves, in intense and peculiar and unreliable ways. Their feelings of worth seem somehow unsteady. Gaudy fantasies of power alternate with those of limp helplessness; self-loathing vies with outrageous vanity.

Adults who happen to be involved either resonate with this self-loving and self-hating, or they don't; they empathize or they remain coldly indifferent. If they resonate, it may be with a mixture of tones, from the highs which approach identification with the "touching" qualities of adolescent narcissism, through the mid-ranges of accepting tolerance tinged with amusement, to the lows of loving outrage. If the adolescent is fortunate, any of these responses, even non-empathic, rejecting responses, may cogwheel into the developmental needs of a given moment. If the adolescent is less fortunate, whether he unconsciously creates his misfortune or simply runs into it, his development may be complicated.

In the course of an investigation into the nature of adolescent narcissism, the psychoanalytic concept "idealization" came under particular scrutiny. In thinking about adolescent idealization, I recalled a striking experience in group therapy 17 years ago (in 1957). At that time I was working with a clinic group of very bright young adolescents. A violent and unexpected crisis erupted, occasioned by the withdrawal of a female observer from the group. Since the crisis and its aftermath were so instructive, at least to me, about transference and countertransfer-

27

ence, I wrote a paper which was published ten years later (Spruiell, 1967).

Like many young therapists, I had at the time two bodies of knowledge, an official set of ideas and formulations and an unofficial set. The official set consisted of an understanding of the basic principles of psychoanalysis, plus the lore picked up from a psychiatric residency. The unofficial understanding could only be dimly formulated, if at all. Mostly, it was rationalized as having to do with my qualities as a "good psychotherapist"; in reality it had to do with ways I used my own personality to respond to the narcissistic needs of my patients in order to "make therapy go."

Luckily, careful notes had been preserved, and on reviewing them and the paper itself, I came to the conclusion that, while there was little to be altered, there were some things to be added. These had to do with the normal narcissism of early adolescents.

NARCISSISM AND IDEALIZATION IN ADOLESCENCE

Idealization, a part of the more general subject of normal and pathological narcissism, was of great interest to Freud. He was particularly concerned with it in several papers (1914a, 1914b, 1921). A. Reich's (1960) and, more recently, Kohut's contributions (1966, 1968, 1971a, 1971b) have proven illuminating, and much of what follows is in obvious debt to them.

All relationships—but particularly those in early adolescence—have narcissistic components. Some friend is apt to be related to as a separate autonomous person and used *at the same time* as a sort of alter-ego and *at the same time* as a sort of externalized ego ideal.* Or another contemporary is apt to be looked on as dirtily sexual, as a degraded version of one's own self, or even as a sort of negative ego ideal. Or an adult, a cause, an ideology, or a group attitude may be used for ego ideal purposes. Or a whole school or town can be seen as applauding one's heroic qualities. Or unknown heroes can be worshipped in secret. The only mixture not easily achieved has to do with uniting erotic and affectionate needs in a single relationship. The point is that the relationships, whether real or fantasied, are complex *mixtures* of narcissistic and non-narcissistic elements; the elements can be separated only heuristically.

In 1914, Freud (1914a) wrote a touching little essay, "On Schoolboy Psychology," regarding the particular idealization of teachers. It should come as no surprise that the same use is also made of youth workers—

---

* For a discussion of the ego ideal in adolescence, see Moses Laufer (1964).

including psychotherapists. As a matter of fact, this tendency to make a hero of the leader helps make individual psychotherapy "work" with early adolescents; coupled with the tendency to idealize peer group standards it also helps group psychotherapy "work." A youth worker or a therapist is apt to lend himself to this use—usually quite unconsciously. As a matter of fact, if there are not *some* tendencies in himself of this sort, the adult is apt to be a failure with young people. Aichorn (1935) emphasized these issues, as did Gitelson (1948).

To some extent, the adult must "let it happen," though if he consciously strives to "make it happen" he is apt to be mercilessly seen through as a "phoney." But this is not all. He who wishes to do well with adolescents must also be prepared to "let it un-happen," to not interfere when he is de-idealized, as inevitably he must some day be.

By the beginning of late adolescence—the age of 16, give or take a year or more—a complex reorganization normally occurs. Ordinarily, there is a coming together of the tender and the erotic (and aggressive) "currents" in the form of romantic love. The boy or girl who is loved seems very wonderful indeed, and the "illusion," in Freud's (1914b) word, develops that he or she is loved for "spiritual" or other "higher" qualities. The loved one is simultaneously idealized and wanted sexually. Now it is not easy to reach this stage, and a tragically large proportion of people are unable to do so. Much of early adolescence is taken up in the reorganizations of mental life necessary in the struggle to achieve it.

The uniting of the tender and the lustful "currents" cannot take place unless the adolescent is able, to *some* extent, to separate from, to become manageably disillusioned with his peer group and with his adult heroes. There is reason to believe that this takes place with the acquisition of an adult body image serving as an organizing influence (Spruiell, 1972). If he is able to accomplish these partial separations, and if his environment cogwheels into his developmental needs, two behavioral changes, among others, emerge: he begins to act in terms of a more or less adult ego ideal and he becomes able to fall in romantic love.

As for the therapist, whatever he does, *he must not interfere* too much with these developmental needs; if he interferes too obtrusively, his cause is lost and the patient is literally better off without him.

It must be apparent that I see nothing "wrong" or "difficult" in the therapist being normally idealized. On the contrary, such a development can become a powerfully useful aspect of transference. But it should also be mentioned that particular countertransference reactions—whether seen in the broad or the narrow sense of the term—are apt to be stirred up. And, as always, the more that is known consciously about these human reactions, the better.

I have been discussing normal and psychoneurotic narcissistic development in adolescence, not pathological narcissistic states. But when these exist—for example, in the form of extreme "pathological idealizations" in perverse or borderline patients—they are apt to serve defensive rather than maturational purposes. As A. Freud (1958) has observed, many attempts at therapy of severely disturbed young adolescents come to grief because the idealizations are apt to be so capricious, premature disillusionments come with such shattering ease, or the demands that the therapist live up to the idealizations are too impossible. Nevertheless, if a satisfactory environment can be provided and acting out controlled, even these patients may respond surprisingly.

CLINICAL EXAMPLE

The group under discussion was unusual in that the boys and girls were of very high intelligence; otherwise it was similar to many other psychoanalytically-oriented groups described in the literature. It had been in existence for three years, but only one charter member remained. The psychologist-observer had attended for about a year; the psychiatrist-therapist, however, was a novice, having taken over from a previous therapist a few months before.

All of the boys and girls were between the ages of 14 and 16. They had been carefully screened to rule out psychotic and sociopathic individuals. A review of the case histories suggests that at least two of the members should have been considered to be "borderline patients."

The observer's role in the group was to remain silent, but not unresponsive. She took notes openly and deflected the many attempts to provoke her into activity. Part seriously, she was often referred to by the boys and girls as the "mother" of the group.

Although often loud and boisterous, the members were well enough behaved and there were only two self-enforced rules: no side conversations and no physical violence. Rereading the notes maintained by the clinic, I was impressed with the number of "id-ish," mostly oedipal, interpretations bandied about. But they seemed to do no harm, and if the group now seems to me to have been handled with a certain amount of naïveté, its ultimate course also seems to document its value to the young people. *How* valuable it was I do not know.

After some disruption, related to the change in therapists, the group had settled down to seemingly active work, and it was in a setting of stability that the observer announced one day that administrative duties necessitated her leaving. A shocked silence followed. It was interrupted by an obsessional boy who attempted to initiate a discussion of splitting atoms. He was ignored, and a number of ostentatious side conversations broke out—about school, football games, and the like. These in turn were angrily quelled temporarily by one of the self-appointed group leaders. The therapist remarked only that the group seemed to be reacting to the observer. A boy commented that "splitting the atom" meant "splitting the family." Another then proceeded to interrogate the observer: Was she married? Was she pregnant? Did she dye her hair?

The therapist attempted to turn the attention of the group to the motives behind these questions, to no avail. There were more and more interruptions. The side conversations assumed a frantic quality. Over the next hour the noise level steadily mounted to deafening levels. A boy started lighting matches, finally managing to ignite a whole book of them at once. "Wants to burn up the place!" shouted one of his friends. With a flushed face still another boy questioned the observer about her sexuality.

The therapist was totally unable to control the accelerating contagion of excitement. Some of the boys laughed about replacing the observer with a "sexy movie star." A picture of one was found in a magazine, ripped out, pinned to the wall, and then pelted by wadded-up paper.

The wildness developed a frantic, manic quality. Girls made paper airplanes and sailed them desperately about the room. The girls alternated between urging the boys on and attempting to protect the observer. One of the girls attempted to offer the observer some chewing gum but dropped it to the floor. Another, swinging her foot, inadvertently kicked the observer. Nobody could stay still. A boy tried to set an eraser afire. Then a wastebasket was lit and the therapist had to intervene to put it out. There was a stench of burned rubber and paper in the smoke-filled room. Finally the session was concluded, although the boys and girls did not seem to want it to stop. Everyone, adults and adolescents, seemed emotionally drained.

What could account for a hitherto tolerably well controlled, "not-too-sick" set of young people becoming not a group but a mob? This kind of reaction to the departure of the observer had not been foreseen. It consisted of a mad celebration of the loss of all restraints to erotic and aggressive expressions—regressive, ambivalent expressions.

It was not a circumscribed affair. Each member later showed behavioral reactions which could be related in individual hours and group sessions to the event. One boy began missing school again and had severe diarrhea and other manifestations of increased anxiety. One of the girls became more isolated and hostile at home, threatening the stability of her whole family. A boy, usually punctual and reliable, missed two successive individual appointments, and seemed distant and depressed. Another girl had such a serious fight with her mother than she left home to live with grandparents. There was only one exception to these negative responses; a boy who had open difficulties with a very paranoid mother became more direct and assertive. In each of these patients, it was possible to relate the loss of the observer directly to the content of the individual session.

The group sessions, too, continued to show disturbance. There were anxious, angry and depressed discussions about acquiring a "talking observer." Some savage squabbles broke out. Stark oedipal anxieties emerged most openly when one of the most anxious boys discussed a man who had literally been castrated.

Interesting as this content was, individual and group sessions began to make it quite clear that the therapist had all along been held in amiable contempt. He was the "newcomer," "too young" to be the "real therapist." For the first time he came to be accused of, among other things, "not keeping good order." Doubts were expressed about whether the group would continue.

It is not going too far to say that the patients were not the only ones narcissistically bruised. The therapist, however, was able to respond by trying to understand his own involvement, and as a result he changed his technique. He gradually became more sure of himself, and by six weeks after the incident the group had settled down and had begun to work on other issues. Shifts in the predominant transferences—and countertransferences—indicated that some mastery of the problems and some working through had taken place. The group went on to become useful for most of its members, and the separations involved later in the individuals one by one leaving the group (a year or two later for most) seemed to occur in a context of real growth rather than regression.

In an earlier paper discussing this group (1967), I analyzed the causes of the group's reaction to the observer's announcement that she would be leaving, causes which in part became obvious in discussions inside and outside the group. To summarize the earlier explanations, it was clear that the observer had been experienced as a much more powerful authority than had been recognized. Her silence, her seeming to grade and judge as she took notes, had invited her being seen as a dangerous enigma. At the same time it could be understood retrospectively that she had been experienced as an object of dependency. The sudden loss of a restricting authority and covert source of gratification initiated fearful, angry and guilty reactions accompanied by expectations of imminent gratifications of unconscious wishes. While each member reacted in his own idiosyncratic way, the confluences of themes were expressed along oedipal lines. These oedipal confluences were what the members had, as a group, most in common; pregenital material and defenses against it, while abundant both before and after, were not considered to be interpretable.

The fact that the oedipal configurations seemed to have a matriarchal quality directed attention toward the therapist's actual behavior. Then it could be understood that the inexperienced therapist had been ambivalently dependent upon the observer for "support." Unbeknownst to him, he had been reacting more like one of the adolescents than as an adult. This relationship between therapist and observer was, however, unstable; it was satisfactory to neither. Ultimately the instability led to the observer's retiring—rationalized as an administrative necessity.

Turning back to the adolescents, there was another commonality: the key members of the group shared a difficulty in that they all had, in actuality or fantasy, powerful mothers seen in phallic terms, and weak or absent or distant fathers. *Thus, the countertransference had complemented the transference.* When the complementarity was disrupted, the group temporarily lost its regulatory organization.

Does anything need to be added, other than details, to the sketch above? That is, can the temporary disintegration of the group into a mob be accounted for solely by a disruption of the group members' customary positive and negative oedipal transferences? By a loss, a destruction of the phallic mother? By a panicky freedom from all parental restraint? By an eventual finding of a stronger paternal set of transferences through the therapist's overcoming countertransference resistances to them?

I believe these things happened, but more happened as well, having to do with the narcissistic aspects of these relationships. Not one of these young adolescents had reached psychological late adolescence. That is, not one had sufficiently freed his psychic organization from attachment to archaic objects and achieved the ego and superego reorganizations to begin to function in adult ways of working or loving. Each was still involved in narcissistic and homosexual object finding; each continued to rely upon "supplies" of functions from adults; each continued a sharp distinction between his peer and his adult world of objects.

In part, the members, to varying degrees, had been involved in transferences—and defenses against them—to both observer and therapist of impulses, feelings and expectations derived from previous relationships with parents. But in part, the observer was *also* invested with idealized qualities—a narcissistic phenomenon—while the therapist was secretly seen in a narcissistically degraded position. Not only did previously hidden reactions to the therapist's "weakness" emerge, but many fantasies about the observer also made their appearance: she was seen as an omniscient judge, the brilliant, self-contained power behind the throne. There were expressions of envious fantasies about her status in life, financial situation, attractiveness, etc.

In these latter terms, the withdrawal of the observer constituted more than a loss of an object; it constituted a narcissistic blow. She had been to some extent the carrier of the remains of some of the lost narcissistic power and grandeur of early life. The observer had thus been a transitional figure, the representation of regulatory functions not yet integrated into the superego. She had carried the meanings of a relationship with a phallic mother *and* simultaneous meanings—normal for the age—relating to a still to be achieved part of the adolescents' respective selves.

In another way there was a narcissistic blow. The observer, with her pleasant attentiveness and careful note-taking, served as a sort of responding screen, a sort of reverberating echo chamber, for the exhibitionistic displays of the young people. The therapist also functioned in this way, perhaps even more so than the observer. It is to be noted that both therapist and observer had regarded the group as quite "special." They had been very proud of the group, and there had been many discussions of "fascinating" things the boys and girls had done and said, of their "incredible insight," of how amusing they were, and the like.

These functions continued the acceptances and empathic responses of the original parents to the boys' and girls' expressions of only partially "tamed" august self-representations. Measured responses of this sort are absolutely necessary in the adult who relates to young people—even if in this case they were perhaps not measured enough. Such responses, and their appropriate modifications with maturation, allow for the ego to become not less narcissistic but more *maturely* narcissistic. A sudden withdrawal, as occurred here, was taken as a rejection; it served as a miniature trauma. The abrupt loss could not easily be dealt with; the group showed a disruption; the individuals not only acted as though they were without regulation, but they regressively demonstrated earlier versions of their own omnipotent and glorious self-representations.

The group was hardy, however, and insisted on the therapist's taking over as an adult who could not only allow himself to be the object of transference impulses, but who could also serve to some extent the transference-like narcissistic functions—both the still uncompleted superego needs and the needs related to the mirroring functions.

I do not mean to imply, of course, that these features were exactly the same for each of the adolescents, or even were present in all of them. There certainly were many complex differences. There was enough commonality, however, to see interactions operating clearly—in retrospect.

DISCUSSION

The clinical illustration makes no pretense to scientifically document the thesis that normal narcissism is a major factor to be considered in any therapeutic approach with early adolescents. No such documentation is needed; the thesis is obviously true. Though obvious, it needs elucidation and expansion. Particularly needed is a sure set of conceptions about narcissism in general and about adolescent narcissism in particular.

Any young adolescent patient relates to a therapist in four convergent but differing ways:

(1) In terms of more or less realistic perceptions of the relationship, considering the individual's age and experience.

(2) In terms of impulses, wishes, defenses, fantasies, and expectations transferred from parental figures of the past.

(3) Similarly, in terms of displacements from parents and others in the present.

(4) In narcissistic terms, dealing with the therapist as if he were a hero who possessed idealized qualities which the adolescent has not yet internalized into his own ego ideal, and/or dealing with the therapist as though he were a sort of parental function admiringly responding to the patient's inner wonderful qualities. In some ways these modes of relating are transference-like; in others they coincide with the realistic aspect of the relationship. Up to a point, these narcissistic transference-like responses are *normal* in the young person; they facilitate growth. Beyond that point they indicate pathology.

The question is not which of the four modes exists, but what combination of the modes exists. The therapist responds, consciously or unconsciously, to each component; if he is aware of these responses they give the earliest indications of the nature of the mix.

The situation is complicated still more with the addition of group therapy. On the one hand, the patient relates to the therapist differently —often astonishingly differently——in the group in comparison to the private behavior of individual sessions. The other group members become a collective third party in the relationship. Accordingly, the relationship becomes vastly more public and either more or less dangerous, requiring different defenses, different behavior. In particular, the role of the therapist as *leader* is much intensified in a group.

On the other hand, in the group the patient reacts in realistic, transferential, displaced, and narcissistic ways to his peers. The transferences and displacements predominantly relate to siblings, although this is by no means always true. The narcissistic aspects of the relationships to the group as well as to the therapist vary in their combinations of "mirroring" and idealizing needs; both of these narcissistic ways of relating become melded with ways of loving and hating based more directly on instinctual motivations. In pairs of group members, the tender and sensual "currents" increasingly combine between defensive breakups. The group stimulates this, since it reduces the threats of strangers, and in a sense siphons off incestuous and murderous impulses onto the person of the therapist, the mutually loved and hated leader.

There is no doubt in my mind that these and other aspects of the group process stimulate confluences of oedipal—and to some extent, pre-oedipal—configurations. At the same time real exploration of pre-oedipal conflicts is discouraged because of the fear of "inner sexuality" (Kestenberg, 1967a, 1967b, 1968), consciously experienced as intensely childish and shameful.

Before further discussion of the relevance of adolescent narcissism, a few words about group therapy are in order. Many psychoanalysts doubt the usefulness of adolescent group therapy on more or less *a priori* grounds. They ask, "How can one keep track of all this when even in individual psychoanalytic work understanding is taxed beyond all limits?" I think the honest answer is that in secondary process terms one cannot— though the research possibilities of understanding by way of videotaping and team-analysis of the data seem promising. But one could also say that parents are unable to keep track of the transferences within the family; yet growth proceeds. Of course, parents do not bring their children up by providing insight but by providing experiences; the important experiences are largely determined by the parents' empathic responses; empathic responses do not necessarily imply insight.

But there is another, related answer. The psychoanalysis of a young adolescent, on the one hand, and group psychotherapy, on the other, are two different things. One seeks intrapsychic reorganization by the analysis, in a setting of great intimacy, of the transference relationship (including its narcissistic aspects) and the defenses. The other seeks to provide a social experience which will aid the adolescent's spontaneous maturation.

However useful adolescent group therapy may be, it must be admitted that there are difficulties inherent in it. If it is a "therapeutic instrument" it is an extraordinarily unwieldy and difficult one. It is not everyone's kettle of tea—witness how few adolescent groups actually exist, and how few therapists continue their youthful enthusiasms for such groups.

If the difficulties can be surmounted, I believe there are great potential therapeutic benefits in group psychotherapy combined with individual therapy (not, *note bene,* combined with actual psychoanalysis, with which it would interfere). The potential benefits include, socially, the provision of a setting for working out problems with peers, the exposure of *some* aspects of the private world to the public world, the experience of looking inwardly, with others, to try to understand motivations, and finally, the awareness that many of the most important motivations operate unconsciously. They include, more inwardly, a setting for the targeting of both transference reactions and normal narcissistic needs—a setting which will hopefully cogwheel into their developmental needs rather than oppose them.

To return to normal adolescent narcissism, it is true that much of what I have to say about it in therapy has to do with familiar admonitions: be tactful; be sensitive. But tact and sensitivity depend upon empathy, and empathy cannot be automatically summoned up whenever needed. There are many things which may prevent us from knowing and feeling what it is like to be a particular young person. Besides the patient's blocks in communication there are our own blocks. These include whatever unresolved conflicts are still barred from our own consciousness. They include unresolved adolescent difficulties and, particularly, narcissistic needs which have never really been transformed, and which continue, though warded off by defenses, within us.

Most young adolescents who come willingly to therapy are caught between very opposing motivations. They have to some extent broken their earlier naïve faith in adults—they have *had* to. But most of them have not lost faith entirely. They are looking to reinvest it more selectively in new adults who they hope can show them, speaking very broadly, how to become men and women. But they must be careful; they must be tentative. Further disappointments might be shameful, even hazardous. Intimacy with an adult flirts with awareness of fantasies of sexuality and aggression with adults, fantasies which are consciously intolerable to most.

So they must be secretive about such things—usually secretive even to themselves. It takes a long time for many a young person to become aware how much he wishes to find an older person who has "made it" successfully into adulthood, how he yearns to believe that an adult could be interested in him, how he reaches out for an adult he thinks to be different from previous models, how he longs for a leader who can show rather than drive, who leads rather than coerces—and how he pines for an older person to side with what he dimly perceives to be the best in himself. And it takes even longer to tell anybody else about it.

How much more secretive a young boy or girl must be about his or her inmost exhibitionistic needs to be admired and adored—approved not for what he or she does but *is!* Even within himself, somewhere, he knows that unrestrained gratification of these wishes would be disastrous for his own autonomy, and disastrous externally as well in terms of the mix of these wishes with wishes to be loved and gratified genitally.

The adolescent must defend himself; he must in open or hidden ways scoff at, deny, make fun of, frighten off, pretend indifference to, withdraw from, hypocritically act as though he were in compliance with, test and test again through provocations, or be silent about such needs and such a relationship. The menace of excruciating shame, mortification, self-doubt, hurt, disgust, and rage is too great.

In a successful, prolonged therapeutic relationship these problems will come to be explored, either openly or implicitly, either overtly or covertly. If the narcissistic aspects of the relationship have been allowed to flower, there will also come a time—usually in mid-adolescence—when the therapist is dislodged from his position in the patient's narcissistic world; he becomes a de-idealized figure, one whose approving functions are no longer so needed. As has already been discussed, if all goes well these aspects of the relationship become partly displaced onto the first genital love relationship, and partly internalized within the patient's own ego ideal and ego. This period, while it may bring up mixed feelings and be painful to both parties—as it is so often between parents and their children—is not hard to understand, at least. In some ways it is a loss, in others an emancipation, both for the young person and for the involved adult.

What, then, are the technical problems in dealing with the narcissistic aspects of the therapeutic relationship?

We must make some basic assumptions: that the therapist is mature enough at least to recognize his immaturities and to be able to prevent their damaging effects; that the therapist should have come to terms with his own narcissistic needs; that the therapist is conscientious and is continuing to examine his own motives; that he is willing and able to call for supervisory help; and that he is willing to retire from a mode of therapy when he clearly shows himself to be unsuited for it.

Actually, no major technical alterations are called for in dealing with narcissistic phenomena. What is called for is a special understanding. The therapist still attempts to develop some kind of contract with his patient. He confines himself to verbal interactions. He listens ordinarily without criticism. He attempts to understand the material and identify the conflicts. He *accepts* the presenting defenses and, behind them, the developing transferences as intrapsychically necessary and potentially comprehensible. He seeks then to open himself to empathically experience the unconscious aspects of the material. He interprets only what is comprehensible and useful to the patient at a given time. If circumstances warrant, he does not hesitate to allow himself to be used as an auxiliary ego or superego.

Misunderstanding the narcissistic aspects of the material or the defenses against these narcissistic aspects often leads to departures from this basic model, whether the departures are conscious and rationalized or consist of alterations of which the therapist is unaware. One has to do with *acting,* or playing a part—or worse, convincing himself of his great "love" or magical "healing powers" or his ability to be a real replacement of parental figures in the past or present. All these reactions betray narcissistic problems within the therapist which need to be recognized and dealt with. They betray an inappropriate idealization of the self, either defensive or simply immature in nature. Or they betray an identification with an idealized picture of the patient; one "loves" and "helps" and "admires" the young person as one wishes one's self to be loved, helped, and admired. These reactions interfere with the therapist's being what he actually is—the adult therapist, who is working with an adolescent patient.

Other alterations have to do with assuming an educational role, or a disciplinary parental role, or a seductive, provocative role, or simply being chronically bored and disinterested, or feeling helpless or even fraudulent as a therapist. Parallel are interpretations of aggression which in actuality are moralistic and hostile in nature, or the early conclusion that the patient is "too sick," or the subtle avoidance of the patient's tendencies to treat the therapist as an alter-ego. All of these reactions betray defensive reactions in the therapist—defenses against either erotic and aggressive derivatives or defenses against unacceptable narcissistic needs.

Kohut (1971a, b) has mentioned several specific rules in treating adult narcissistic personalities, and I believe they apply also to normal narcissistic phenomena in early adolescence. They include the avoidance of early interpretation of the patient's needs to idealize or seek an alter-ego, the avoidance of intellectualized interpretations, and the avoidance of overly strict adherence, to technical rules which are appropriate for adult neurotic patients, i.e., in regard to formality, distance, the ideal of confining the interventions to interpretation, the suppression of non-verbal spontaneity in the therapist, refusal of gifts, etc.

If therapy in early adolescence, whether individual or group, has not interfered with normal processes of growth, the separation which takes place in mid-adolescence requires no special techniques. The therapist must in *some* senses relinquish the patient at that time. If continued treatment is indicated, the question is whether the patient can safely use a vacation period and whether the continuation in late adolescence should be with another therapist who has not shared an actual part in the young person's development.

SUMMARY

In this paper, I have deliberately and artificially separated out narcissistic phenomena shown by more or less normal and psychoneurotic young adolescents in order to demonstrate their importance in therapy. I do not believe that the narcissistic phenomena can be *actually* separated from love-hate phenomena involving other people as truly independent objects. There is always a combination. But the narcissistic aspects have not been stressed in the literature, and it is my belief that the misunderstanding and consequent mishandling of normal narcissistic needs and defenses against them account for a sizeable number of failures in the treatment process.

REFERENCES

AICHORN, A. (1935). *Wayward Youth*. New York: Viking Press.

FREUD, A. (1958). Adolescence. *The Psychoanalytic Study of the Child*, 13:255-278.

FREUD, S. (1914a). Some reflections on schoolboy psychology. *Standard Edition*, 13:241-244. London: Hogarth Press, 1961.

FREUD, S. (1914b). On narcissism. *Standard Edition*, 14:67-102. London: Hogarth Press, 1961.

FREUD, S. (1921). Group psychology and the analysis of the ego. *Standard Edition*, 18:69-143. London: Hogarth Press, 1961.

GITELSON, M. (1948). Character synthesis: the psychotherapeutic problem of adolescence. *Amer. J. Orthopsychiat.*, 18:422-431.

KESTENBERG, J. (1967a). Phases of adolescence—I. *J. Amer. Acad. Child Psychiat.*, 6:426-465.

KESTENBERG, J. (1967b). Phases of adolescence—II. *J. Amer. Acad. Child Psychiat.*, 6:577-614.

KESTENBERG, J. (1968). Phases of adolescence—III. *J. Amer. Acad. Child Psychiat.*, 7:108-151.

KOHUT, H. (1966). Forms and transformations of narcissism. *J. Am. Psychoanal. Assoc.*, 14:243-272.

KOHUT, H. (1968). The psychoanalytic treatment of narcissistic personality disorders. *The Psychoanalytic Study of the Child*, 23:86-113.

KOHUT, H. (1971a). *The Analysis of the Self*. New York: International Universities Press.

KOHUT, H. (1971b). Thoughts on narcissism and narcissistic rage, presented as the Brill Lecture, New York Psychoanalytic Society.

LAUFER, M. (1964). Ego ideal and pseudo ego ideal in adolescence. *The Psychoanalytic Study of the Child*, 19:196-221.

REICH, A. (1960). Pathologic forms of self-esteem regulation. *The Psychoanalytic Study of the Child*, 15:215-232.

SPRUIELL, V. (1967). Countertransference and an adolescent group crisis. *Internat. J. Group Psychotherapy*, 17:298-308.

SPRUIELL, V. (1972). The transition of the body image between middle and late adolescence. In *Currents in Psychoanalysis*, I. Marcus, ed. New York: International Universities Press.

3

The Structure and Setting of Adolescent Therapy Groups

MAX SUGAR, M.D.

Some adolescents walk in and out of treatment quickly. Every youngster seen is not a candidate for analysis or intensive group therapy. The youngster may be functioning all right, but comes upon a situation he is unable to handle. That problem may require him to have brief or lengthy help with the issue; thus many of the youngsters seen need only a couple of sessions to unhook some barrier (Winnicott, 1973). If the youngster has another troublesome problem, he may return for further brief or long-term therapy, as needed. If he once has a successful therapeutic encounter, whether in one or ten sessions, the positive effect remains, and he knows that if he needs more help, he may return. This may reduce some suspicions and feelings of inadequacy, while raising some feelings of self-esteem.

The adolescent who may benefit from intensive group therapy is the youngster who is having some chronic problem. The youngster who needs only brief therapy will not be around long enough for the therapist to involve him in a group. Group or intensive individual therapy may be needed for the youngster who gets stuck in some unproductive behavior, who continues having symptoms or the same misbehavior that got him into difficulty, or who makes repeated academic miscalculations.

The adolescent who needs therapy may be more comfortable if treatment is possible in a therapy group, where he sees other people who appear to be in a similar mess. It is natural for adolescents to form peer groups for a variety of reasons, including sexual development needs, the reduction of anxiety, separation from parents, and testing of personal independence. The younger adolescent, especially, may find comfort in being with a group, which may reduce some of his inner pressures related to distrust and fear of adults, and sexual pressures including masturbatory impulses.

The 12- to 14-year-olds are preferably placed in groups with their own sex. There is cultural pressure to get involved with the opposite sex, but at that age interest in the opposite sex is not intense. The inclination is rather to avoid the other sex because of revived oedipal conflicts, with incestuous fears and wishes. These young adolescents need to figure out what is going on within themselves before they get involved with those strange creatures of the opposite sex. Thirteen- and 14-year-olds form gangs naturally; the boys play various athletics, such as baseball, football, or pool (parlor or pocket), and the girls become involved in groupings to learn how to use make-up, how to dress and impress boys at a distance, how to get along with parents and teachers, and how to get out of doing homework and other things.

The middle phase of adolescence is less likely to be as clear-cut in terms of homogeneity, although there is still a clear tendency for groupings which involve both sexes more than in the earlier years. There is anxiety about this, masked by diffidence or bravado, with possible efforts to escape from the anxiety by use of counterphobic measures with the opposite sex. They are making efforts to cope, usually becoming more involved with dating, perhaps, or going out in groups of couples.

The grouping becomes increasingly heterosexual through the late teen years, and the institutions adolescents are involved with, such as school, communes or work situations, lend themselves to group formation.

The middle and late adolescent groups often include both sexes. Group therapy composition should be related to the patient's needs, age span, psychosexual levels, levels of integration, positive attributes, diagnoses, and nuclear conflicts. Adolescents' groups, particularly in the early adolescent years, should be organized so that there is no more than a three-year gap between any two members. Otherwise the youngsters cannot function effectively in the group, since their developmental tasks are too disparate to allow them to really understand one another and work effectively. A 13- and a 15-year-old can work well together. A 15-year-old may conceivably work with a 20-year-old, but less effectively than in a group with other 15-, 16- or 17-year-olds. I try to organize groups so that the early adolescents are from 12 to 14 years of age, and the middle ones from 15 to 17 or 18. The late adolescent group can comprise those from 17 or 18 to 21 or 22.

The youngsters start questioning one another with "What grade are you in?" "What school are you in?" "How old are you?" by which they check out the other person, comparing and contrasting themselves with one another. If they cannot find something in common, whether it be the same school grade or similar interests, they have more difficulty forming a group. This need for "common interests" may be related to problems with communication of personal and intimate feelings which transcend interests.

If a group is formed with six or eight compulsive boys, all of whom are making A's in all classes and are therefore having no trouble at school, but whose parents are worried because they only stay at home and study, worrying about passing tests, it might be a rather cumbersome group. On the other hand, a grouping of eight or ten schizophrenics, aged 14, will provide a different kind of quandary.

Another problem arises with some patients who at 18 or 20 are so anxious about themselves and their impulses that they simply cannot function well in a mixed group. Their anxiety is at such a high level that they perspire profusely as soon as they see someone of the opposite sex. This kind of youngster may not be suitable for a mixed group.

The clinical picture of each youngster should be viewed as a distinct and individual matter and the selection process carefully thought out before assigning him to a group. Each potential member has to be thought of in terms of how he is going to fit in with A, B, C, D, and so on, in various ways. The level of maturation, judgment, reality testing, their usual defenses, the state and ease of regression, the integration they have achieved, and the threats to their integration all have to be considered.

A guidance or mental health clinic group needs other considerations as well, which are different depending upon the setting of the group—in private practice, a university clinic, or a state hospital. Each of those settings has special requirements that need to be met, and if they are not considered, much is missed or neglected that is important to ensure the proper structure of the group and promote its ultimate success.

An institution that has an oppositional attitude to group therapy makes it difficult to arrange groups, or to meet with patients for evaluation for group therapy. A common practice in such a setting is that instead of selecting suitable patients for group therapy, patients that are felt to be untreatable individually are referred for group therapy. The patients, therefore, are not selected carefully or grouped according to their needs, but are put into a group because of expedience. If this kind of arrangement is followed, the staff members soon become frustrated because they do not have suitable group composition or successful groups. A successful group does not necessarily mean that everybody in the group gets "cured," but that the group becomes a cohesive, therapeutically functioning group. If it is not set up for that, the staff eventually gets frustrated, and ends up having group after group dissolve after a few sessions. Then they feel, like the administration, that group therapy does not have much value. In that case, the administration has proven its point "scientifically."

Patients confined in a state hospital often feel that they are coerced to attend therapy sessions. Such patients may have distorted and magical thinking and feel, for example, that unless they attend, their food will be poisoned, or they will have to stay longer in the institution. Here the problems may be related to the fact that the setting offers an aura of confinement in which the patients expect to be regimented. They may view the therapy session as a kind of torture chamber. Here the therapist must be on the alert for and deal with this kind of paranoid thinking and distortion. Otherwise his interpretations, although skillful and precise, may never help the group to develop a therapeutic working alliance.

In some ways this can be easier to handle, perhaps, than the situation in private practice in which patients come voluntarily. If they do not want to enter the group after being carefully prepared, they can walk out and never return. This, too, may frustrate the therapist, leading him to limit himself to individual work rather than attempt group therapy. He may need to evaluate dozens of people before selecting one group of ten that will constitute a suitable, potentially viable group. On the other hand, if the patients have no choice in the matter, the therapist can expect to face all the problems incident to coercion. In an outpatient clinic, a university clinic, or in a state hospital, there are usually more patients waiting to be seen than there are available staff, and the therapist may therefore consider forming a group for them. In private practice many adolescents do not stay very long, and if they are available for a group, not all of them may fit in the group being planned. Thus, the problems of setting up such groups in private practice seem to be more difficult in some ways than in an institution.

In an outpatient group, the groupings can be made on the basis of the particular needs of the patients or the first ten patients can simply be assigned to one group and the next ten to the next (Burdon and Ryan, 1963). The latter approach may work, but there seems to be a greater possibility of success with a group that is carefully selected. But even in the optimal setting, once the adolescent group therapy starts all sorts of contingencies may arise. The parents may interfere because they feel that the family's private life or their child's escapades may become public news, even though they are in the confidential files of this outpatient setting. Or teachers and principals may interfere by telling the child, "I don't think you can go off today because you're missing too much school. You had better stay here. You can't attend the group." It is therefore important for the therapist to establish positive rapport with parents and school personnel to gain their cooperation for the youngster's benefit. Sometimes this becomes a contest to the parents or the school as they may feel that their role somehow is threatened, and that the therapist will be able to do magical things for the child where they have failed. If cooperation is not established, the youngster will begin missing appointments, being late, having to leave early, or having contingencies arise that interfere with his being in the group.

Some outpatient groups function well with very disturbed youngsters, such as aftercare groups for those who have been in state hospitals. These adolescents are followed up in group sessions, which are held every two or four weeks. This is not brief therapy, because it may go on for years. But this frequency may be all that is needed to allow them to touch home base to check out a few things and to help them with further integration. This is one kind of group that has been successful for some youngsters, by offering support through the adolescent years and helping them towards better integration via peers, which may be less threatening than it would be individually.

The outpatient adolescent group with neurotic and characterological diagnoses may meet on a regular basis every week, for an hour or an hour and a half, and do quite a lot of good work. In my own practice, I handle intensive group therapy by a number of arrangements with which the youngsters must agree before we proceed. I insist upon: confidentiality about the identity of group members and content of sessions; avoiding socializing with group members while members are in the group; a commitment to remain in the group for at least six months; and individual responsibility for one's attendance.

These matters are also explained to the parents, when the fees are arranged. When the youngster pays, even if partly, the fees are discussed with the adolescent. Administrative matters about the group should be managed by the therapist, whether in a private practice or clinic setting.

A problem that often comes up is the unscheduled extra group meeting, when the youngsters have a difficult time ending their session and feel they have to continue it outside. It may be due to excitement or contagious anxiety leading to some temporary cohesion or acting out. When adolescents have gotten together afterwards, they will later bring in the material, once they understand how and why the group arrangements work to their benefit. At the next session they may be quite hostile, ambivalent and disagree with the conditions, but they know that we have an agreement that they made voluntarily for their own benefit.

Part of the agreement is that they do not have any extra-group contact; if they do see one another outside of the group, it should be purely by accident, and then they should attempt to bring in their feelings about it to the next group session. I explain that they are going to have all sorts of feelings about seeing one another outside after they spend all these intense hours over many weeks or months with each other. Thus I let them know that this may happen in advance, and discuss what they may do about it. Outside contacts that occur are usually brought up fairly quickly, although it sometimes takes weeks or months.

There was one youngster who was extremely withdrawn and very threatened by the thought of being with any people, and particularly with girls his age. After he had been in individual treatment awhile, he entered a mixed group, and there he became a little less frightened of girls. At the same time he started making some arrangements to meet girls through some of the male friends that he had made by that time. One of the ways he checked himself out about girls was to meet with one of the girls in the group on the basis of altruism, a quality he had in abundance. He considered this girl so downtrodden and poor that he felt moved to buy her good records so that she might hear the latest good music, and to take her to his home to listen to the records properly because he had a stereo while she had only a portable hi-fi player. Then she appeared so hungry all the time that he invited her home for dinner with his folks. He chose a girl who was "weak" and therefore less threatening as a potential castrator. Finally, these outside contacts came up in the group where they were viewed as acting out and discussed in detail. By that time he had some reduction of anxiety about females, his sense of maleness was confirmed and he was able to discontinue the acting out.

The setting is an important communication given by the therapist to the patient. In Chapter 4 on "Group Therapy for Pubescent Boys with Absent Fathers" it is apparent that when the stimuli of toys and noise-makers were removed, the group changed in its goals and functions. This change in direction eventually led to another level of object relations and ego functioning. Berkovitz (1972) noted that some therapists provide candy, cokes and cigarettes for a variety of adolescent therapy groups to decrease anxiety. These provisions may compensate for a deprivation, but unless the group members have such a deprivation syndrome (Winnicott, 1958) and the group is arranged specifically to deal with that need, applying this arrangement routinely to interpretive therapy groups may be nontherapeutic. It may actually aid resistance in that the provision of gratification may seem to be a bribe. Similarly, if the group is left uncertain about how many members it has, since the number may be between 12 and 16 because of variable attendance (Ackerman, 1955), the patients get the message that their presence is not of great concern. Then their attendance may become variable. By contrast, if each member is told before entering the group that there is a maximum number of patients (8 or 10 or 12) and their attendance is important and their responsibility, regular attendance usually ensues.

SUMMARY

Therapy groups for adolescents offer some particular enhancements for some youngsters to have therapy. These involve such matters as their conforming to peer values and trusting them more than adult persuasions. Attention to the specifics of cooperation with parents or guardians, diagnosis, age and setting is of prime importance to deal with varieties of resistance that may impede forming a group and later having a working alliance within it. Differences in arrangements abound between private practice, a clinic and a state hospital.

When group therapy is arranged for adolescents for ancillary purposes and individual therapy is the primary approach, then relaxed arrangements about composition, number and structure may offer a social practice arena. Where group therapy is the primary, or coeval, therapy, then attention to diagnosis, number of patients in the group, their attendance and balancing become more crucial matters for explicit arrangements.

When a therapy group becomes important to a youngster, his attendance is usually quite regular. The therapist can utilize the above described principles to develop that sense of group importance.

REFERENCES

ACKERMAN, N. W. (1955). Group psychotherapy with a mixed group of adolescents. *Int. J. Group Psychother.*, 5:249-260.

BERKOVITZ, I. H. (1972). On Growing a Group: Some Thoughts on Structure, Process, and Setting. In *Adolescents Grow in Groups*, I. H. Berkovitz, ed., pp. 6-28. New York: Brunner/Mazel.

BURDON, A. P., and RYAN, W. (1963). Group Therapy as Primary Treatment in an Outpatient Setting. In *Current Psychiatric Therapies*, Jules H. Masserman, ed., 3:229-233. New York: Grune and Stratton.

WINNICOTT, D. W. (1958). The Anti-Social Tendency. In *Collected Papers: Through Pediatrics to Psychoanalysis*. Pp. 306-315. New York: Basic Books.

WINNICOTT, D. W. (1973). *Therapeutic Consultation in Child Psychiatry*. New York: Basic Books.

4

Group Therapy for Pubescent Boys
with Absent Fathers

MAX SUGAR, M.D.

A significant relation between parental deprivation and incidence of emotional illness has been noted in several reports (Dorpat et al., 1965; Greer, 1964; Nichol, 1964; Heckel, 1963; Gardner, 1956; Brown, 1961; Beck et al., 1963). Whereas the effect of maternal deprivation has often been implicated in the development of serious psychopathological states, effects of paternal deprivation have received comparatively little attention (Bowlby, 1951; Spitz and Wolf, 1946; Provence and Ritvo, 1961; Provence and Lipton, 1962; Wheeler, 1956), and treatment has received even less.

Gregory (1965) suggested that the identification model provided and the control normally exercised by the parent of the same sex are more crucial in preventing delinquency among children than is any aspect of the relation with the parent of the opposite sex. McCord and associates (1962) noted that boys developed feminine-aggressive behavior, accompanied by intense sexual anxiety, if the father had been absent when the child was between the ages of six and twelve years. The father's absence correlated especially well with gang delinquency. In the study by Wylie and Delgado (1959), mothers sought psychiatric help for fatherless boys only in times of crises, under external pressure, usually from schools. The boys were difficult to treat because the mother could not control their aggressive behavior. Among prominent observations were the following: the boys were doing poorly in school; half of them were enuretic; a fourth of them were encopretic; the fathers were considered bad by the

Reprinted with permission from *Journal of the American Academy of Child Psychiatry*, Vol. VI, No. 3, July 1967.

mothers, the boys were similarly viewed by the mothers and were pressed to assume the father's role in the home; the relation between mothers and sons was highly sexualized and hostile; half the boys slept in the same bed with their mothers; and the mothers were closely tied to their own parents, often living in the same home with them.

Green and Beall (1962) described a type of paternal deprivation in boys in which the father is psychologically remote from his son and physically absent from home. These boys also had academic or behavioral problems at school, as well as physical and other symptoms.

Pollock (1962) observed that for boys the loss of the father in the oedipal period is more crucial than at any other time. He concluded, however, that the effect of the loss of either parent depends on the age of the child at the time of loss, the sex of the child, the pre-existing difficulties, and the reality situation of the child survivor.

STRUCTURE OF THE GROUP

In a therapy group of pubescent boys the outstanding common feature was some degree of paternal deprivation. This paper reports on some of the significant aspects of their dynamics and treatment.

Over a period of twenty-seven months, twenty fatherless boys from varied socioeconomic levels and between the ages of eleven and one half and thirteen years were treated in an open group for periods ranging from two to fifteen months. Not more than ten boys were in the group at one time. The group met first in a clinic setting (The Louisiana Evaluation Center for Exceptional Children), and during the last nine months, the group was seen in a private office practice. Six months after group therapy for the boys began, some of the mothers entered a mother's guidance group in the same facility. Their group terminated after eight months. In the private practice setting, the parents were seen individually only, at approximately monthly intervals.

The boys were brought to the clinic by their mothers, on the advice of school officials or friends, because of difficulties in school performance and behavior. The diagnoses included neurotic and adjustment reactions, behavioral, character, and schizoid and passive-aggressive personality disorders. In seven instances, the father's absence was absolute and attributable to suicide, death, divorce, or desertion. The separation had occurred during preschool years in five and in the latency age in two. The other thirteen fathers had been absent irregularly because of divorce, long working hours, alcoholism, or hospitalization for emotional or physical reasons.

COURSE IN THERAPY

During the first few sessions, the boys were anxious about the strange new situation. They resembled an activity group of latency children; they paired rapidly, played peek-a-boo, made models, banged on a pounding board, and smeared art materials all over the blackboard and on drawing pads. When anyone asked a question or tried to talk, the noise was accentuated by pounding, shouting, and jostling of chairs. The therapist tried to minimize the anxiety by making supportive or interpretive remarks or by moving close to the youngster who seemed excessively anxious or threatened.

When the therapist announced in the second session that the fourth session would be postponed for a week, the boys became noisier and shouted. This reaction, which was partly an index of hostile attachment to the therapist, reflected their separation anxiety and reaction to loss. The third session was marked by increased noise and a general tendency toward obstreperous and destructive behavior. The therapist had to control and limit the boys actively. They seemed to be saying, "Don't leave us; we need you to help us and control us." In the fourth session, they showed considerable anxiety and anger in their play. When their behavior was interpreted as related to the interruption in therapy the week before, they appeared to retaliate by defiantly isolating the therapist. They played poker, drew and colored pictures, crawled into bookshelves, and generally absented themselves from the therapist. They seemed to be playing hide-and-seek, wanting the therapist to find them if they were important enough to him.

In the fourth and fifth sessions the theme of abandonment was also displaced to the adventitious circumstance of a pigeon's nest with eggs which was within reach of the group room. Several of the boys wanted "the eggs to hatch at home, because the pigeon is not there, she's left the eggs" or because "the pigeon deserted the nest."

Efforts to control bullying and hostility among the boys by interpretation and by pointing out the democratic process and majority rule were unsuccessful. The bullying represented part of a power struggle with authority in general, and of a test of the displaced mother's-therapist's authority in the group. The boys treated the therapist as they did their mothers, with hostility and defiance. He had to be firm and set limits when they seemed on the verge of hurting one another by shoving swivel chairs around. They took turns being "slave" and "master" in a game involving mastering passivity and reversing roles: one boy sat in a swivel chair and another rolled him around as directed by the occupant. Passive aggressiveness was also evident when the "master" relinquished responsibility for bumping into the other boys who happened to get in the way as the "driver-slave" pushed the master's chair.

Mark, the tallest boy, tried to handle his feelings of inadequacy by his usual bullying. The group reacted with hostility and defiance. The ensuing fractious remarks and efforts to hurt one another were interrupted by the therapist. The boys pointed out that Mark's flaunted knowledge of poker and other card games was false; one boy beat him regularly after first being somewhat threatened by his allegedly superior knowledge. Competitive efforts for leadership continued, with challenges, denials, and threats.

Ned, who felt he could not compete at all, was extremely anxious most of the time and often tried to cling to the therapist. When not using these techniques he withdrew by reading out-of-town newspapers or doing his homework during the session. Often he indicated his displeasure with the group by complaining that it was not working the way he had hoped and that no one listened to his problems. He tried to irritate the group by such comments as, "Nobody is saying anything," "Nobody has any problems here." "What are we trying to do?" or "Nobody is listening." His stated wish to be more involved in therapy increased the scapegoating directed toward him, which, in turn, fulfilled his masochistic needs.

The group's continued hostile dependency on the therapist was manifested in many ways. When the boys felt anxious or threatened, they turned to him, but resisted his interpretations by silencing him with noisemaking or shouting or by pairing in card games or other play activity. Some of them asked for advice and suggestions in their games, whereas others tried to test and provoke the therapist. He was cast in the transference role of mother, and each complained of the others as siblings and wished to have the exclusive care of the mother-therapist; when their wishes were not fulfilled, their behavior usually became defiant and hostile. Some boys tried to become the therapist's favorite while testing to find out if they were acceptable to him. This behavior seemed to be related to their concern about being acceptable to mother, and to the fact that father had apparently not been acceptable to mother.

Toward the end of the ninth session, the therapist introduced refreshments in an effort to supply an organizing focus of communication and communion. This was also based on Winnicott's (1958) idea of treating the paternal deprivation through provision of some actual supplies and comforts by the therapist. It seemed to help the boys abandon some of the regressive behavior through a fulfillment of oral needs and demands and led to more discussion, especially of sexual matters. By the twelfth session, with the sharing of food and words, a good deal of cohesiveness had occurred, sexual excitement had increased, and homosexual feelings had become somewhat uncomfortable. Some of them ran to the bathroom in follow-the-leader fashion, or in pairs, for brief periods. The boys were involved at several levels of feeling but they tried to avoid expressing any friendly feeling verbally. They maintained distance through hostile exchanges, including swearing, verbal attacks, and squirting soda pop on one another as well as onto the walls and floor. This behavior was interpreted to them as a masturbation equivalent as well as an expression of hostility toward the parent-therapist. Attempts at fighting were interrupted by interpretations, persuasion, or physical intervention by the therapist.

In the fourteenth session, Ned complained of not feeling well and of being tired from working hard in his summer job with his father. In reply to questions, he explained that his mother had just delivered her tenth child, "a baby boy." Ned's hostility toward the baby and his simultaneous denial of the baby's existence reflected his intense sibling rivalry, jealousy, and hate. He identified with his mother and her confinement by lying down on the couch, and with the newborn baby by lying down in the group-family, inviting the therapist-mother to care for him.

At the next session, Ned mentioned that his mother thought he had stolen money when he believed he had taken some of his own money. The group challenged his defensiveness and denial of guilt. It was explained to him that the incident indicated his anger toward his mother and his wish to take something from her, or even actual guilt for having taken the money. The group decided spontaneously to set up a "court." They elected a judge, prosecuting attorney, and defense attorney, with Ned as the defendant in the "Case of Stealing Money from His Mother," with credits and references to television's Perry Mason. Ned immediately wanted to phone his mother from the therapy room, to find out whether she had found her money. The group accused him of calling for other reasons. They paraphrased the therapist's remark that perhaps he thought he was going to miss some attention by not being at home. Ned's attempts to deal with his new sibling helped the other members understand their own sibling rivalries, jealousies, and hates.

The therapist's approaching summer vacation heightened the boys' anxiety, dependency, and hostile feelings. They reacted intensely as if fearing they were being deserted by their mothers for siblings or by fathers for various reasons. They scrambled for possession of the swivel chair; which symbolized leadership and prestige; its occupant was considered the favorite child in the group.

During the summer vacation, some members dropped out and new ones entered the group after sessions were resumed. As the group adjusted to the loss of old and the arrival of new members, they verbalized as they had previously about girls and about their problems at school with teachers and at home with family members. The group became more cohesive, and affectionate bonds grew among the members as they delved into feelings about girls. They began again to engage in slightly disguised homosexual play, such as sitting in one another's laps or stretching out on the couch so that one's head was in another's lap, or two of them sitting together in one chair. During an episode of the latter type, Mark seated in Evan's lap said, "This is really togetherness."

Some of the boys noted that their noisemaking was used to interrupt talk. The therapist reinterpreted their fear of expressing feelings and covering it with noise. He indicated the connection with changes, such as his vacation, or absent, departing, and new members, as well as with fears of telling secrets to adults.

Mark's behavior progressively reflected the shift to verbalization. He became more comfortable, felt less inadequate, and could use verbalization instead of activity to express his feelings. He now felt that he could use his mind and could see progress in his schoolwork. Some of the others who had been in a subgroup or in a paired situation with him followed his lead and began to shift similarly. Mark discussed girls and his previous antisocial behavior and contrasted himself with Charles, who remained antisocial.

During the week of the twenty-fourth session, some of the mothers joined a guidance group directed by a female social worker. The boys had mentioned this fact in connection with anxiety about exposure. They seemed now to derive satisfaction from the knowledge that their mothers were being taken care of and they therefore did not simultaneously have to depend upon and look after their mothers.

By the twenty-sixth session, the boys began to discuss openly their feelings about fathers. Kenneth was trying to deal with his father's suicide, whereas Joe and Ned were trying to deal with hatred of authority. In defense against their anxiety there were comments about relative sizes, strengths, physical masteries, and skills. They were struggling for favorite sibling position in face of fear of exposure as they dealt with the absent father. Their hatred and fear of authority now seemed related to the dreaded fantasy of his return.

The group was now well into the middle phase. The members had also begun to deal with sexual feelings openly. They feared each other and the therapist less, and their view of the therapist shifted from the ambivalently needed, hated, desired mother to the needed, but hated, absent father.

When Vic and Charles dropped out of the group at their mothers' request, the group attacked the therapist for getting rid of them. The unpredictable attendance of Vic and Charles for several months previously was similar to their fathers' unpredictability in being at home. The vehemence and intensity of the continuing attack seemed related to displacement and reversal of feelings about the absent father. It was their own absent, rejecting, deserting father whom they were attacking. But the transference continued to be mixed; the therapist was still viewed partly as a mother-figure who had inexplicably removed the father.

In contrast to previous hostile, negative discussions of heterosexual matters, their discussions now indicated hatred of mother and sister mixed with positive feelings toward other girls. For some weeks, the hatred of mother for having destroyed the father was displaced again upon the recent dropouts.

By the thirtieth session, the group had moved further toward an understanding of father and persons in authority. In response to several situations, they again set up "court" and elected officers; this arrangement permitted verbalization, and no punishment was carried out. They were symbolically displacing the mother from her role of final authority, identifying with the father, and possibly trying to show what a father should and could do. Some felt guilty about their displaced hatred of father, and several times the most outspoken member stayed away the following week after outbursts had occurred toward the therapist. During several "court" sessions, the boys discussed various matters related to guilt. On occasion, they had the therapist participate as a witness because he supposedly knew all about certain allegations made by one member about another. This may have been an ambivalent expression of friendliness toward the therapist and identification with the aggressor, as well as an effort to use authority to hurt their rivals.

The boys were now better able to deal with and to talk of fears of and hostility toward parents, reaction formations, projections, passive-aggressive maneuvers, murderous impulses, and sibling hatred. When feelings causing increased anxiety became too troublesome for them to handle verbally, however, they reverted to noisemaking by pushing chairs around, swiveling around, shouting, and banging on the pounding boards. In the thirty-fifth session, the therapist removed all toys and other objects that invited regressive behavior or discouraged verbalization. Only one chair for each person was kept in the therapy room. When Ned asked the therapist why he had removed the objects, the defensive use of these objects to avoid feelings was again interpreted. They turned to discussion of their good report cards and of some of their angry, destructive, anti-social acts, such as breaking street lights and windows and stealing knives from stores. The admissions led to more talk about hatred for their fathers. Kenneth, especially, hated his father and, for the first time, told of mistreatment by his stepfather. It was explained to him that he was apparently using the mistreatment to justify his antisocial acts. Others were stimulated to confess past antisocial acts.

The early, strong latent homosexual attraction between Larry and Kenneth was so disturbing to some of the others that they verbally at-tacked them. This reaction seemed to be an angry denial of their wish for reciprocal affectionate feelings from their absent fathers. Their pairing gradually began to give way, however, with Kenneth's general improve-ment and his increased ability to deal with his anger, depression, and identification with the therapist. Larry became upset over Kenneth's academic and behavioral improvement and continued his acting out against authority in school and outside.

Although discourse about their feelings was now easy, when anxiety became too high for them, they retreated. The group theme was pre-dominantly their desertion by the absent father—their anger and depres-sion over the desertion and their fear of the omnipotent authority whom they could not see.

When it was learned that Ned and his mother had discussed their group sessions with each other, the boys became angry with him for having violated their confidence. They decided to try Ned a second time in "court." Ned was fearful of and cried about being rejected, ostracized, and perhaps harmed. The group pronounced sentence of "No more Cokes for 50 to 200 weeks." Some of the others had also broken the group confidence, however, and Ned was merely being used as a paranoid target. When they tried to do him bodily harm, the therapist assumed the role of the protective father and prevented it.

They were now dealing with broken confidences, difficulties with au-thorities, and loss of respect for parents. In subsequent weeks they pro-gressed to include feelings about the father who disappointed them and about the adults, including the therapist, who made mistakes. Later topics included methods of retaliation against parents for disappointments and unfairness, such as failing in school, throwing eggs against school windows or in auto gas tanks.

By the end of the first year when two new members came to their first session the group discussed horror movies, science fiction movies and books, girls and hatred of girls. Kenneth's remark that Vic now wanted to return to the group was followed by noisemaking, foot banging, angry remarks to the therapist, and attempts to use toys again. Efforts to discuss the meaning of this behavior led to verbal attack on the therapist for removing the toys sometime before: "You can do this, you're the boss," "It's your right, you're in charge," "We were making too much noise so you had to take the games away," "You were jealous of us playing with toys 'cause you couldn't play with them."

When asked if they wanted to hear the therapist's reason, they said yes. As soon as he began to speak the babble of noise, foot banging, and angry remarks recurred. When the therapist stopped talking, they stopped noisemaking and laughed. The angry interaction was allowed to continue until it spontaneously ended. Then the therapist interpreted their angry reaction to him as displaced hostility from the newcomer.

When the therapist took over the mother's group in the week of the forty-second session, the boys became anxious about possible interchange of information about them between their mothers and the therapist. Their anxiety was expressed in both verbalization and action during the sessions. On one occasion, Kenneth lay down on one of the chairs with his feet on another chair and made disparaging remarks about the position of the female during intercourse. Guns and other weapons, destruction, masturbation and intercourse, maleness, and the ability to deal with women and to stand up to father all became major topics. The boys' progress was indicated by their ability to verbalize defenses against castration anxiety instead of using action. The decreased defensiveness was manifested by their revealing their dreams.

Ira, who had slept with his mother until recently, began a discussion of dreams: "I dreamed of being in an elevator which was held by a single cable, very rickety, and the elevator was going very fast, way up and up. The walls of the elevator were very far away from me, and it seemed that we were about to hit the side and it was very dark. I was very frightened and the elevator just kept coming up and up and up." The therapist remarked that this certainly would be a frightening feeling and asked if the other members had not also had frightening thoughts, feelings, or dreams. All had had dreams of falling, being stabbed or otherwise at-tacked, or killed, some dreams were in color and some were in serial form. None of the dreams was interpreted at this time, but they were used rather as a means of ventilation and of sharing anxiety about loss of control to ego-alien tendencies by day, and to dreams and nocturnal emissions by night.

In the forty-seventh session, it was apparent that some of the hostile responses by certain members were attributable to the awareness of certain qualities in themselves similar to those in others. Each of them was a product of an undesirable father who did not want children and who therefore deserted them through divorce, suicide, or absence for long hours at work. Some mutual antagonism was based on having had similar fathers, each stirring up uncomfortable feelings and memories in the others on this basis. As these hostile projections were interpreted, further feelings about closeness, affection, heterosexual and homosexual feelings and drives were brought up. The boys were now able to accept and deal with these despite initial intense anxiety.

The group members defended themselves against intensified castration fears by discussing size, strength, weakness, and fears of being hurt. Their wish to be protected and cared for by the therapist, as if he were their father, was clearly expressed by Ira's remark, "We are Dr. Sugar's nuts." They and the therapist belonged to each other, they felt.

When Larry and his mother discontinued therapy, the others, especially Kenneth, reacted strongly. He had been alienating himself from Larry for several months, having discovered that they were no longer doing things similarly. Now, however, he felt guilty that the separation may have caused Larry to leave the group. This reaction was interpreted as a displaced wish fulfillment and as retaliation for his father's suicide. Kenneth experienced a period of open mourning and depression, feeling that he was responsible for his father's death, just as he had been responsible for Larry's leaving. Kenneth feared that he would also commit suicide. He talked about his parents' separation and the difficulties that followed. His ambivalent wish and fear of being separated from his twin were also related to his feelings about Larry's departure.

Evan detailed his accidentally blinding a boy with a BB gun two years before and the pending lawsuit. A discussion followed about sexual inter-course with many questions—who had done it, how it is done, and how pregnancy occurs. Having intercourse with an unknown "hole in the rubber" was one of the methods of getting girls pregnant.

Then fears of women, fears of being hurt, and the folklore of harmful consequences of masturbation and intercourse followed. With a great deal of laughter, Kenneth now revealed that a year ago he had had an unsuccessful operation for an undescended testicle resulting in his having only one testicle. He said, "I wouldn't waste the other one on girls. I'm never going to have babies." He went on disparaging himself despite clarification about physiology from the rest of the group and the therapist, and compared himself unfavorably with his twin brother especially in athletics, particularly baseball. He then described being hit by a baseball in his remaining testicle after the operation, the agony he experienced, and how he "chickened out" from baseball that season. He resumed playing baseball the following season (since in group therapy) and the night before he had "hit a homer with a man on."

The rest of the group became very anxious in relation to this material, and most of them responded with personal anecdotes about their agony when they had been hit in the testicles, and the use of steel protectors in boxing, football, etc.

Following this, speeds in running races were compared, and several members tried doing handstands, hand holds, judo holds—a defensive maneuver to demonstrate potency and deny their castration fear.

In the late months of therapy, the boys functioned more satisfactorily at school and had few problems with authority generally; parents and teachers were not complaining as before. Dynamic changes also became evident in their group behavior. Mother was discussed as a hateful object, but with some wistfulness in phrasing or tone. They became concerned about their appearance, and hair styles acquired great significance, whether "flat-top," "duck-tail," or "Beatle" cuts. Madras shirts, blue jeans, and other popular wearing apparel occupied their attention, especially differentiation of "Frat" from "Hood" styles of clothing.

Positive association with peers, in contrast to the previous, almost exclusive, monotonous, hostile, and destructive attachment to authorities, was manifested by their joining baseball teams, school bands, informal combos, and other extracurricular groups. As their interests spread, they indicated that they preferred these activities to being in the group. Interest in and fear of girls and "making out" preoccupied them, as well as masturbation and specific matters of sexual behavior. They brought up such problems as how to talk on the phone to a girl and what to do about disagreement with parents over "phone hogging" and mixed parties. As they became more peer-oriented, they became less involved with the therapist and less angry at him. They were better able to deal with interpretations, associations, and dreams.

When the therapist tentatively mentioned the matter of dissolving the group, the boys had mixed feelings about it. In some ways, their transference was still intense and for the most part positive. The majority seemed to have undergone a structural change; they had abandoned their numbing defenses and were moving on with the usual adolescent trials, errors, and experimentations. They were also anxious to go to trumpet lessons, baseball games, or other activities, but still did not miss group sessions. When, after a month or so, a termination date was definitely set for three months later, there was a reactivation of fears, anger, and sadness about loss of and rejection by the therapist-mother-father. Whereas this reaction was vivid, it was not unvarying and not as intense as earlier reactions had been to separation for vacations or departure of members from the group. At the first mention of termination, Kenneth said, "You don't like us and want to get rid of us." Later he reminded himself and the therapist of "how we used to squirt pop on the walls and how you used to shout at us." Hostility to authority was interpreted, and it was explained that since they no longer had a need to do such things, he no longer had to shout at them.

The termination was similar to that with other patients; patients and therapist had mixed feelings of gladness and sadness. The boys needed reassurance that the therapist would see them again if they ever needed help and that they were now ready to go on their own.

DISCUSSION

Anna Freud and Burlingham (1943, 1944) posit an intense and persistent attachment to a fantasied father constructed out of whatever ephemeral tissue is available. Blos (1962) noted that "adolescent boys often transfer the need for passive dependency to their father and the more strongly the passive need is felt—as in overindulged or severely deprived children—the stronger becomes the defense against it by rebellious and hostile actions, and fantasies."

The need for the pubescent boy to remove himself from mother has been noted by Anna Freud (1958), Fraiberg (1955), and Blos (1962). The boy's need for "object removal" is related to the necessity to give up incestuous objects and to avoid fusion and emotional surrender. However, this process may be interfered with by the mother's defensive maneuvers toward the boy. When she has lost her husband and has an overcathexis of the child, she may perceive and react to the boy's separation at adolescence as another rejection by the husband.

The initial hostile and rebellious symptoms of the boys in this group may have been related to a search for a father, that is, for someone to help them. Their behavior may be viewed as an effort to avoid fusion with mother and deny passive dependency needs, as well as to separate themselves from incestuous objects. In addition, they might have been acting out their mothers' views of fathers and expectations of all males. The learning difficulties may have similar bases; learning successfully was considered feminine by these boys and, conversely, being a poor student was equated with masculinity. Their need to defend against being, or becoming, a girl was related to their sexual confusion. Indeed, learning from a female teacher (whom they all resisted) was equated with dependency gratification from mother.

Absence of the buffer aspect of the normal biparental situation and synchronization and dosing of oedipal experiences (Neubauer, 1960) prevented development and resolution of the oedipus complex, with its resulting identification with father and development of a suitable super-ego. The absence of the father also inhibited normal aggression toward, and emancipation from, the remaining parent (Eisendorfer, 1943). Eisen-dorfer described a split, severe, archaic superego and an immature and excessively dependent ego in his two female patients with missing fathers; both were highly narcissistic, had poorly coordinated egos, and were incapable either of adequately controlling their id impulses or of dealing with their environment. Similar pathological ego and superego functions were observed in varying degrees in the boys in the present study.

The therapist's difficulties in working with adolescents have been described by Lampl-de Groot (1960). Anna Freud (1958) noted the adolescent's lack of interest in the past and in the analyst; his concern is solely with the present. Fraiberg (1955) commented on the difficulties a female therapist has in treating early adolescents, especially girls. Early adolescence is characterized by a tendency to gang formation and socialization of guilt (Blos, 1962). Group therapy with a male therapist appears to offer an approach, especially for early adolescent boys, that fits in with their spontaneous tendencies and needs. The group initially focuses on the here-and-now; being able to share and socialize guilt without punishment fits their needs. Having a male therapist reduces some of the early resistance and is less threatening, since it removes them from mother and mother-substitutes and provides a male figure with whom they can identify and about whom they can have fantasies. The therapist who works with adolescents, especially in a group, needs a flexible approach that can shift from interpretive to supportive work. He must be willing to set limits and controls actively as well as to use the environment whenever possible. Ultimately the therapist's skill with adolescents, and not his sex, determines his effectiveness.

The early sessions of group therapy in the present study were marked by dependent, defiant, hostile, rebellious behavior toward the therapist, whom the boys at first unconsciously identified with mother. The intensity of their transference to the therapist as mother was evident in their reaction to the first break in regularity of sessions. The anxiety seemed to be related to an exaggerated need for mother as the remaining parent and to anger at the mother-therapist for leaving them. Adolescent boys with absent fathers seem to be characteristically mother-oriented rather than peer-oriented.

The unresolved dependency and other oral conflicts were manifested in early activity and play, which duplicated the behavior engaged in with mother and mother-substitutes. Provision of limited direct oral gratification during the sessions permitted eventual verbalization of some of the conflicts and led to discussion of the postponement of tension discharges by action, which disrupted the cycle of inhibition-defiance-guilt-anxiety.

Although the adolescent in treatment does not usually become intimately involved with the therapist initially (Fraiberg, 1955; A. Freud, 1958), his later transference is intense, especially if he has an absent parent (A. Freud and Burlingham, 1943, 1944; Eisendorfer, 1943; Keiser, 1953; and Meiss, 1952). I have observed this type of transference in children and adult patients who have an absent parent, and particularly in children in residential treatment. The intense transference was evident in this group whether the therapist was viewed as mother, father, or other imago, positively or negatively. The cause may be overcathexis of the remaining parent and idealization of the absent one, or fear of loss of the remaining parent. Due to its being so intense and complicated, a much longer time than usual was needed for some resolution of the transference. Again, in the termination considerable extra time was required for the group to work through their reactions to termination as there was some recurrence of the intense transference feelings.

The *truly* fatherless boys had less conflict than those with *relatively* absent fathers. In Neubauer's (1960) patient, "the father's influence proved more pathological than the remaining parent; in addition to his pathology, the timing of his visits, rather than the timing of separation, intensified the already existing developmental conflicts." An irregularly present father seems to be a particular threat to the child because he cannot mourn for him and work through the absence (Keiser, 1953). Such a father creates more of a problem than a dead or otherwise absolutely absent father because the child does not know how to deal with unpredictability. Keiser (1953) described a girl with a superego defect from not having had an opportunity to desexualize the oedipal attachment; her father was neither a dead parent whom she could mourn and finally forgive, nor a present parent with whom she could have a real relation, with its attendant frustrations and ultimate resolution of the oedipus complex.

Bringing the mothers into therapy, and later into a group with the sons' therapist, symbolically re-created the original family for the boys and allowed buffering and synchronization of oedipal experiences. This arrangement provided further stimuli for dealing with fantasies of the lost father and of the therapist as father; for working through the oedipal conflict, superego difficulties, and identifications; and for helping with the need for "object removal." In the process, castration anxiety increased, and was accompanied by defensive, tough male talk and homosexual play. With mother in a group, her cathexis and seduction of the son were reduced, and he could become aggressive and separate from her. The boy was also relieved of the obligation of being his mother's protector, since the therapist was caring for mother, and mother was learning to care for herself.

The dynamic change in the boys was especially evident in the "courtroom" episodes and in their responses to loss and arrival of new group members. The initial "court" was autocratic. After the election of court officials, the elected judge meted out sentence. This procedure apparently represented the boys' fantasy of what the active, powerful, fearsome, phallic mother could do. The judge embodied feelings of an external, punitive, primitive force which they could not control, and the sentences, although not enforced, were harsh judgments indicative of a very severe, archaic superego. The "court" did, however, mark a forward shift in superego and ego function, in contrast to the previous deficient internal controls. Early "courts" were often identified with the *Perry Mason* television show, in which the defendant is usually innocent. In later episodes, the whole group contributed to judgments, and the court shifted to trial by a jury of peers. The shift indicated the presence of an internalized superego: guilt without actual punishment, postponement of gratification of sadomasochistic impulses, and increased responsibility for their acts. In ego terms, it indicated that "object removal" was occurring.

The theme of violating confidentiality with mother pointed up their guilt about incestuous wishes, the desire to separate from mother, keep their own secrets, and set limits and controls for self, with less need for punishment by mother (which had previously given oral and sadomasochistic gratification). The judgment of no refreshments for "50 to 200 weeks" for violating group confidence also disguised the wish to be fed and taken care of for a long time by the therapist-father-protector. The "court" may therefore be introduced by the therapist deliberately, as a technique in latency and adolescent groups.

When Vic and Charles left the group at their mothers' requests, the group had an intense mother-transference reaction as if the mother-therapist had eliminated the father. This exposed them to the guilty fear that the powerful, punitive, active mother might do this to them as well. Thus Vic and Charles were viewed as part father and part dependent-and-helpless self. The arrival of new members was reacted to partly as to separation and death. The response to new members was related to this as well as the usual anxiety about exposure and strangers, and sibling rivalry. Later, when other members dropped out or new ones came in, the reactions of sadness or anger were not as intense or prolonged as responses to earlier departure or arrivals—another reflection of their modified superego and ego functioning.

The group initially reacted to the therapist as to mother, wishing to test and provoke the therapist-mother and concomitantly to have him set limits for them. In this phase, the rapid and intense pairing may have been another aspect of the maternal transference, expressed in clinging to a peer. After the initial phase, in which the mother transference to the therapist was intense and prolonged, interpretive, supportive, and active therapy enabled the group to move gingerly into the middle phase, in which they began to verbalize more, used their spontaneous "court" to solve certain problems, and began to view the therapist as the absent father. Some identification with the therapist and subtle work on their ties to mother were in progress. The next direction of major work was the mourning for the lost father, with shifts in reaction to the therapist, first as the lost father, next as the rejecting mother, and then as substitute father.

Some obvious homosexual defenses appeared in sequence, initially as a defense against their incestuous wishes and castration fears, and then as a narcissistic defense as they moved on to "object removal" and gave up efforts to have mother. The therapist and other group members were then viewed as father or brother, and the attachment was a tender, passive, homosexual one. From this point on, the group themes were mainly related to shifting ties, to experimentation of various sorts with peers of both sexes, and to dealing with sexual and aggressive impulses. The boys seemed to have resolved some of their atachment to mother, revived and mourned the absent father, given him up, formed new ties to a father-substitute and given him up, worked toward giving up some of their previous defenses, and achieved some "object removal" and sexual identity. They were entering nonincestuous object relations and were then in the middle phase of adolescence.

SUMMARY

Twenty pubescent boys with absent fathers and with the initial complaint of academic failure or behavioral problems, or both, were treated in an open group for periods varying from two to fifteen months. The entire study lasted twenty-seven months. The multiple problems of this group are considered from the standpoints of setting, composition, and management. Common to all the boys was a father who was absent—by death, divorce, or lack of interest. The group was further characterized by marked sensitivity to separation, intense transference, and an almost exclusive relation with maternal authority rather than peers. The choice of a male therapist was fortunate.

Early in treatment, the therapist was viewed partly as a nonthreatening, supportive mother-figure, and this role was the positive aspect of the patients' attitudes and transference reactions. Regression created behavior similar to that in activity groups.

As the group progressed therapeutically, their predominant attitudes and behavior changed so that the transference to the therapist as a father-figure became more positive and the mother transference became minimal. The shift was reflected in their functioning as an interview group, without games, toys, or behavior of an activity group. It allowed stimulation and support of their moves into positive male identification and resolution of some preoedipal and oedipal conflicts.

Therapy gave these boys the opportunity to deal with conflicts before solidification of pathological defenses. Without therapy, the possibilities of fixation continuing through adolescence may have led to other, more serious neurotic or delinquent manifestations. After receiving help in dealing with the loss of father, they were able to work through some resolution of the oedipus complex in therapy. In so doing, they attained a suitable superego and could therefore proceed with the usual problems of adolescence.

REFERENCES

BECK, A. T., SETHI, B. B., and TUTHILL, R. W. (1963). Childhood bereavement and adult depression. *Arch. Gen. Psychiat.*, 9:295-302.

BLOS, P (1962). *On Adolescence: A Psychoanalytic Interpretation.* Glencoe, Ill.: Free Press, pp. 72-74.

BOWLBY, J. (1951). *Maternal Care and Mental Health.* Geneva: World Health Organization Monogr. No. 2.

BROWN, F. (1961). Depression and childhood bereavement. *J. Ment. Sci.*, 107:754-777.

DORPAT, T. L., JACKSON, J. K., and RIPLEY, H. S. (1965). Broken homes and attempted and completed suicide. *Arch. Gen. Psychiat.*, 12:213-216.

EISENDORFER, A. (1943). Clinical significance of the single parent relationship in women. *Psychoanal. Quart.*, 12:223-239.

FRAIBERG, S. (1955). Some considerations in the introduction to therapy in puberty. *The Psychoanalytic Study of the Child*, 10:264-286. New York: International Universities Press.

FREUD, A. (1958). Adolescence. *The Psychoanalytic Study of the Child*, 13:255-278. New York: International Universities Press.

FREUD, A., and BURLINGHAM, D. T. (1943). *War and Children.* New York: International Universities Press.

FREUD, A., and BURLINGHAM, D. T. (1944). *Infants Without Families.* New York: International Universities Press.

GARDNER. G. E. (1956). Separation of the parents and the emotional life of the child. *Ment. Hyg.*, 40:53-64.

GREEN, M., and BEALL, P. (1962). Paternal deprivation—a disturbance in fathering: a report of nineteen cases. *Pediatrics*, 30:91-99.

GREER, S. (1964). The relationship between parental loss and attempted suicide: a control study. *Brit. J. Psychiat.*, 110:698-705.

GREER, S. (1964). Study of parental loss in neurotics and sociopaths. *Arch. Gen. Psychiat.*, 11:177-180.

GREGORY, I. (1965). Anterospective data following childhood loss of a parent: I. Delinquency and high school dropout. *Arch. Gen. Psychiat.*, 13:99-109.

HECKEL, R. V. (1963). The effects of fatherlessness on the preadolescent female. *Ment. Hyg.*, 47:69-73.

KEISER, S. (1953). A manifest oedipus complex in an adolescent girl. *The Psychoanalytic Study of the Child*, 8:99-107. New York: International Universities Press.

LAMPL-DE GROOT, J. (1960). On adolescence. *The Psychoanalytic Study of the Child*, 15:95-103. New York: International Universities Press.

McCORD, J., McCORD, W., and THURBER, E. (1962). Some effects of paternal absence on male children. *J. Abnorm. Soc. Psychol.*, 64:361-369.

MEISS, M. L. (1952). The oedipal problem of a fatherless child. *The Psychoanalytic Study of the Child*, 7:216-229. New York: International Universities Press.

NEUBAUER, P. B. (1960). The one-parent child and his oedipal development. *The Psychoanalytic Study of the Child*, 15:286-309. New York: International Universities Press.

NICHOL, H. (1964). The death of a parent. *Canad. Psychiat. Assn. J.*, 9:262-271.

POLLOCK, G. H. (1962). Childhood parent and sibling loss in adult patients: a comparative study. *Arch. Gen. Psychiat.*, 7:295-305.

PROVENCE, S., and LIPTON, R. C. (1962). *Infants in Institutions.* New York: International Universities Press.

PROVENCE, S., and RITVO, S. (1961). Effects of deprivation on institutionalized infants: disturbances in development of the relationship to inanimate objects. *The Psychoanalytic Study of the Child*, 16:189-205. New York: International Universities Press.

SPITZ, R. A., and WOLF, K. M. (1946). Anaclitic depression: an inquiry into the genesis of psychiatric conditions in early childhood. *The Psychoanalytic Study of the Child,* 2:313-342. New York: International Universities Press.

WHEELER, W. M. (1956). Psychodiagnostic assessments of a child after prolonged separation in early childhood. *Brit. J. Med. Psychol.,* 29:248-257.

WINNICOTT, D. W. (1958). The antisocial tendency. In *Collected Papers: Through Pediatrics to Psychoanalysis.* New York: Basic Books, pp. 306-315.

WYLIE, H. L., and DELGADO, R. A. (1959). A pattern of mother-son relationship involving the absence of father. *Amer. J. Orthopsychiat.,* 29:644-649.

5

The Organization of an Adolescent Unit in a State Hospital: Problems and Attempted Solutions

ADOLFO E. RIZZO, M.D., ABEL OSSORIO, Ph.D., *and* LEONARD SAXON, M.A.

INTRODUCTION

In dealing with an adolescent population in a hospital center, we have to remember that they are too old to be spanked and unsuitable for analysis. Here lies the conflicted situation that has to be faced by the administrators and therapists: the institution of controls (spanking) versus the effectiveness of more orthodox types of treatment (therapy). At this point everyone embarks on the journey of seeking a solution. But which one? We will start with the distribution of "advice" if this can be forgiven: the solution is conditioned by, and almost unique to, each center.

The basic structure described below can be adapted to other types of residential centers and could include a larger "ecological system" that Auerswald (1969) described as a future treatment modality for children and their families. But, as in any other process, experiences from other attempted solutions are valuable.

Our particular setting was a pre-adolescent and adolescent unit, on the grounds of a state hospital (St. Louis State Hospital), with a capacity of 65 beds. The population served was mostly from an urban area, up to age 17, and with diagnoses including antisocial, severe neurotic, and psychotic adolescents. The staff population also varied from highly motivated individuals to others with a "just passing by" attitude. All of the staff personnel recruited to work at the adolescent unit and those transferred from the main hospital were "volunteers." This alone was not a sufficient guarantee that they would be able to function adequately. Therefore, it was arranged that if any of them felt distressed in the new situation, or if the director felt a change in staff would be beneficial, staff members could be transferred back to their old jobs without a negative entry on their records as a job failure. This was necessary on only two occasions. Besides the in-patient service, the unit served outpatients and satellite clinics in other areas of the county, took part in school and court consultation, and trained residents, fellows in child psychiatry, and other professionals.

The total analysis of these factors, including the physical set-up, determines the particular configuration of treatment plans. Our task was the creation of a specialized unit within the hospital structure that would be specifically designed for the treatment of the pre-adolescent and adolescent patient. Our first task was to study the actual structure of the organization, that, as was pointed out by Kahne (1959) is "a legitimate and fruitful concern of psychiatrists and social scientists."

PROBLEMS

The unit was initiated on a single ward with 20 girls ranging in age from 12 to 17.

After approximately one year of functioning, this unit was moved to a separate building with a 65 bed capacity for boys and girls. In order to develop a treatment program for this population in a systematic manner, we were forced to examine in detail the organization and administrative structure of the hospital and the problems which this posed for the development of a dynamically oriented milieu ward. In the light of this analysis we then had to develop a set of working principles whereby these problems could be minimized within the unit itself, and between this unit and the remainder of the hospital.

One of the basic problems of hospital organization which we felt inhibited the development of a milieu program was the organization of the hospital into what Jules Henry (1957) has referred to as a system of "multiple subordination."

> Systems of multiple subordination are being rapidly eliminated from task-oriented organizations in Europe and the United States. The essential characteristic of systems of multiple subordination is that the worker is subject to several supervisors. In the process of eliminating multiple subordination from modern industry, it has been found

that inefficiency and emotional stress develop as a systematic consequence of such structures, because the worker has to give heed to several bosses at once.

In a modern hospital, systems of multiple subordination still enjoy an exuberant development. Thus charge nurses are subordinated to nursing service, to nursing education, to administration, to the medical departments, and to the numerous physicians who leave orders for their patients. Staff nurses and even aides may also be subject to multiple subordination, for although orders from the higher echelons are supposed to be transmitted through the charge nurse, they may be given directly to her subordinates who are in the grip of multiple subordination.

We have many examples of the effects of this type of organization upon the actual operations of the hospital. An example of interlocking and conflicting group systems which need to be understood can be seen when one tries to set up the daily activities of the patients. Which professional group is more important and higher on the totem pole of treatment procedures? The individual therapists? The educators, etc.? The situations for conflicts here are too many to detail and are familiar to anyone dealing with this system. But on many occasions the patient may just sit on the ward while the staff involved continues the feuding.

In general, the effect of a system of multiple subordination is to release anxiety-hostility conflicts in the individual staff members. The resulting insecurity then leads to attitudes of passivity and excessive dependency in work situations. Individual initiative is inhibited because of the possibility that it may place the individual in conflict with divergent expectancies of various supervisors. The outcome is limited utilization of therapeutic potential, the abdication of responsibility as described by Kahne (1959), and the development of informal information organizational systems within the lower echelons.

These informal systems consist of patterns which are developed on an unofficial basis by personnel in attempts to change or improve their position within the hospital, and also to cope with the problems with which they are presented. This can be done, for example, through bypassing immediate authority, undermining it, forming cliques, and passively resisting instructions. At higher levels, anxiety is a typical response to any deviation from standard procedures, such as emergencies or incidents of "patient misbehavior." A usual solution is to try to find a loophole in the organization or to place blame on those who supposedly failed in their responsibilities. Administrative situations of this type are likely to result in the creation of new rules, operative procedures and functions designed to prevent their recurrence.

A brief example of the inability of administrators in multiple subordination systems to take immediate action and of the potential for acting out by the personnel within such systems can be seen in the following. Information leaked to the lower staff members about a plan for "mass" elopement by several of the boys who were in residence in one of the adult wards of the hospital at that time. Because of conflicting views by personnel regarding treatment (permissiveness), and lack of controls (punishment), the information took several hours to pass up to the proper superior with the aid of written memos. By the time that the higher echelon staff therapists (doctors) were notified, just before a case presentation, the patients had already eloped. This provoked a host of reactions from the administration. The staff members dealing with adolescents were blamed, and they were sent by the superintendent with the order to "pick up your boys" over a hundred miles away—a so-called "learning experience!" A new set of restrictions was devised to prevent such occurrences.

This incident indicates how "following the book" may serve to express resentment and hostility by personnel who are not involved in a therapeutic approach with this type of population. These functions and rules are often not sufficiently defined and frequently conflict with those previously established. They also tend to create jurisdictional problems concerning their supervision. The net effect is to increase confusion within the treatment operation itself, through the development of an increasingly complex bureaucratic set of procedures.

The system presents a situation in which everyone's initial effort is toward doing "the best for the patient," and the final outcome is that everyone tries to get "the best for oneself" and to "be safe." The need to "be safe" leads to a literal interpretation of instructions, failure to report unpleasant situations or, conversely, to exaggerate failures of procedures which are not accepted. This can be illustrated by the following incident: on one occasion the physician was called by the parents of a youngster who had complained to them that some older patients had forced him to participate in homosexual activities. When further inquiries were made, it was found that many of the night shift aides were aware of these activities but never reported them. In this case not reporting an incident could be utilized to protect oneself from censure by superiors and/or to compete for status vis-à-vis other hospital elements. In the meantime the patient is lost sight of to a disturbing degree; personnel become increasingly involved with "administrative problems" as opposed to the treatment functions for which they are best employed. Therapeutic action with respect to disturbing "incidents" (elopement, destruction of property, suicide attempts, etc.) is usually not possible in the above-described multiple subordination system. As a patient's behavior is debated among multiple supervisors, it becomes an isolated and disturbing "incident," a "problem" to the smooth operation of the hospital, to be controlled or prevented, and the context which gives meaning to this behavior is forgotten.

An example of these problems may be seen in how an incident was handled on an adult ward with adolescent patients. A rather well-built 15-year-old boy with a personality disorder became belligerent for several hours, until he struck an old deteriorated patient. The personnel took no action but to immediately notify the clinical director. The treating physician, whom they resented because of his rather authoritarian attitude toward personnel and his refusal to accept their previous requests for restraints, was not notified because he "couldn't be found." He first learned of the incident when he was called by his supervisor. The reaction of the administration was to return the patient to the Court because he was untreatable, against the recommendation of the therapists.

FACTORS INVOLVED IN A THERAPEUTIC MILIEU

Faced with the problem of organizational structure and its attendant problems, we hoped to develop in this unit a new kind of structure, a treatment team in which the widest possible diversification of skills, information, and knowledge would be possible. Kahne (1959) said, "Specialization and division of labor tend to blind participants to the total picture." We hoped to replace the confusion about responsibilities with a system of intercommunications in which all of the individuals in the treatment team would have more self-responsibility, greater flexibility of role, freer access to authority, and a more consistent environment in which better human relationships could emerge. The fact that this was a new unit opened the possibility of cutting down the traditional bureaucratic procedures which develop in large organizations.

The organization that we hoped to develop was designed to handle the problems of staff turnover. Experiences reported by others working with adolescents units led us to anticipate a large turnover in personnel— more than is usual in general hospitals—because of the demanding nature of the work. Turnover in personnel tends to disrupt the continuity of the treatment program. More importantly, it prevents the development of staff cohesiveness within the team which is a necessary condition for a milieu program. This problem can be approached in two ways. First, one can provide maximum job satisfaction and emotional support to staff so that the need to leave may be attenuated. Second, one can try to mitigate the disruptive effects of turnover if it does take place.

Since disruption is maximal whenever a program is dependent upon a few "key people" who possess a monopoly of the skills and knowledge which the treatment team requires, our effort was directed towards lessening the dependence of the treatment team upon a few "experts" through appropriate training programs. Raising the general level of skill among all personnel would help to attenuate a great deal of the frustration which is involved when a person is given a task for which he feels inadequately prepared. At the same time, the development of a diversity of skills and the ability to function in a variety of roles with respect to the patient broadens the interest of the staff in the overall program. Each staff member then has maximum opportunity to identify with the total treatment goals of the unit. The training of staff with this goal in mind must be experiential in nature; didactic teaching or verbal communication alone by an "expert" is insufficient.

Such training and learning can be brought about only as staff members function in different role relationships in close collaboration with each other, so that a common appreciation of the problem and its therapeutic meaning can be learned. The development of the treatment program then utilizes the creative potential and energy of the entire staff, rather than being "carried" by a single person. Flexibility and change are possible, since the staff is not bound by the particular approach of a single expert.

We hoped that this distribution of responsibilities and the resulting intercommunication would lead to the development of an esprit de corps among the unit staff. This, in turn, would provide the emotional security necessary for the individual member to tolerate loss of autonomy, subject himself to criticism from within and without the unit, and make it possible for him to place treatment needs of the unit above personal status involvement within his own disciplinary hierarchy.

A necessary prerequisite for the development of this team spirit is an increased flow of communication among all levels of staff. We have found that communication is most difficult when information has to be passed upward by subordinate staff, and there are several reasons for this difficulty. First, there may be taboos with respect to certain kinds of occurrences. For example, incidents of homosexual acting out among patients may occur which are extremely difficult for nursing personnel to report upward. Sometimes information is withheld about occurrences which are perceived by staff members as representing some failure in duties and there is an inhibition about reporting this for fear of censure. At still other times, especially when the social and professional distance between one staff member and another is perceived as being very great, information is withheld because of attitudes of hostility toward someone with whom communication is difficult. The individual staff member may feel that what he has to report will not be considered important. Where attitudes of passive hostility towards the authority figure are present, the withholding of information may be designed to create difficulties for a particular superior. In still other cases, a staff member may identify too closely with a patient and withhold information in order to "protect" the patient from "unjust procedures."

Creating an atmosphere in which free communication is possible among all levels is probably the most important function of the psychiatric director of the unit. If the director himself possesses the personal qualities which make the staff feel that he is completely accessible, this will have a great influence on the development of this atmosphere. His function as coordinator of all treatment activities carries with it the responsibility of tolerating information which might be critical of him and his philosophy. The capacity of the director of the unit to adopt this kind of task orientation to problems of communication in turn influences the staff to adopt a similar attitude. There is then less danger that subordinate staff will develop modes of response characteristic of the hierarchical type of organization which we have described above.

Another crucial function of the unit director is that of dealing with the problems which exist in developing appropriate relationships between the unit and the rest of the administrative structure of the hospital. Generally, difficulties in relationships between the unit and the rest of the organizational structure of the hospital have two forms. In one sense the hospital reacts to the unit in much the same way that society reacts to the delinquent youngster. Secondly, the unit is identified with "problems," with acting-out behavior which may threaten the relationships of the hospital to the community, and in general as a chronic irritant to the hospital community, making what seem to be inordinate demands for privileges and facilities. One consequence of this situation is that relationships between the unit director and the hospital administration are likely to involve a considerable amount of friction which must be handled tactfully and constructively.

Another focus of conflict centers around the relative degree of "control" which the individual department or disciplinary hierarchy exercises upon the particular staff member within the unit. Control in this sense refers to the extent to which the department or disciplinary head determines the specific functions and activities of a member of that discipline who is assigned to the adolescent unit. This type of determination of functions and roles may conflict with what is perceived by the director of the unit as necessary for that particular treatment program. The staff member is then caught between the demands of his disciplinary superior and the demands of the unit. Particularly, we have found, perhaps by tradition or by the nature of the responsibility, that relinquishment of control is most threatening to the nursing group (Jones, 1953) and to the physician. Without resolution of this problem, the treatment goals of the unit cannot be carried out.

STAFF ORGANIZATION

When all of the above considerations were analyzed, it became a question of how to make the variety of personnel into a functioning unit. Here, we departed from the usual method of in-service education, which is characteristic of mental hospitals (Kahne, 1959). We decided the first phase should be the "grouping" of the staff in functioning units.

To that end we obtained the help of experienced leaders in group training whose functions were to advise, observe, and "trouble shoot." This phase took several months of intensive group training. Working teams were organized with members of all the different professions. The groups were given specific tasks, such as the design for admission of new patients and the integration and responsibilities of the different subgroups. The groups slowly began to deal with their own anxieties, differences, and confrontations between their ideals and the total hospital community.

An example discussed was the question of the expectation by the administration that these would be "verbal" groups and not "acting-out" groups. In the past there had been some groups with a high incidence of destructiveness and aggression due to a more "permissive" type of therapist. This is a real source of conflict as Kraft (1971) stated, "Therapists in these circumstances face the question of control each time the group meets." Each leader's own resolution of the conflict of control determines whether he can continue with the group or will undermine the group's existence. The solution sometimes requires a change of leader.

The process of growth in the groups was reflected in the shift of attitude toward the unit leader, from disorganized passivity to rebelliousness, to contending that the leader was a tyrant, to complaining that the leader was not directing them, to the final phase of separation-independency. The training which took place here was of utmost importance for the operation. Besides the given tasks, many other aspects came out, such as the differences in roles given to the different professionals. The "higher" the status (physicians), and less secure in their position (residents in training versus staff), the more difficulties there were in giving up roles. By the end there was a more realistic exploration of their anxiety regarding new functions, and acceptance of new roles of others.

This phase of the organization was terminated after the groups were functioning and expressed the wish that this particular training be terminated. Looking back with the insight given by time, stopping the training proved unwise as there were training placements continually coming in without basic training, and because leadership should have been maintained to sustain cohesiveness and stimulation. The need to maintain an outside consultant is obvious. After the example of belligerence mentioned above, a consultant continued coming to the unit once a month for several more months, but unfortunately later on it was not possible to continue this due to a change in the financial arrangements. The outside consultants functioned importantly as observers, intervened when needed at times of group immobilization and taught group techniques.

ATTEMPTED SOLUTIONS: STRUCTURE AND FUNCTIONS OF GROUPS

The unit was organized in terms of a number of interlocking groups designed to provide:

(a) A milieu that would take into account and facilitate the working through of the normal developmental struggles of the adolescent.

(b) A therapeutic milieu in which a maximum of interaction could be obtained among staff and patients.

(c) Maximum communication among all levels of staff and patients.

(d) A context within which staff could be trained, with new roles and functions defined.

(e) Sufficient flexibility to allow for the introduction of new approaches.

The following is a graphic representation of the characteristics of these groups and their functions.

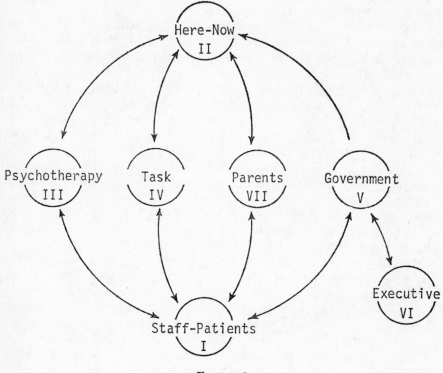

FIGURE 1

The basic "social unit" of the therapeutic community consisted of a patient-staff group (Group I). The entire ward was divided into such groups with each patient and staff member assigned to one of these groups. For example, one unit might consist of 7 patients, one or two nursing personnel, a psychologist, a social worker and psychiatrist. We had several objectives for this structure. First, we wished to take advantage of the need of adolescents to seek identification with a peer group, and to use this motivation as a therapeutic influence. The more dominant-authoritarian models that pretend to offer ideas for identification are really not operant in the present culture. A. Freud (1969) pointed out that "At present, though, this solution is comparatively rare. More frequent is the second course where the peer group as such or a member of it is exalted to the role of leadership. . . ." The present structure offered the opportunity to use these forces in a constructive way as the adolescents were able to play their own roles.

The group functioned in terms of norms to which the individual members would conform to protect the individual patient and which served as a buffer in some of his relationships with the staff, and as an instrument whereby increasing responsibility for conduct could be placed not only upon the individual patient, but upon the group as a whole. These groups would function, therefore, at different levels that would take into consideration the individual patients' working in their "inner world of conflicts" and "the relationship to the external world" (Deutsch, 1967).

The effectiveness of the group setting can also be seen in moments of crisis. One situation arose when a patient eloped one morning after he had returned from a weekend pass. The patients in his group were quite concerned about what he might be doing during this elopement as they were aware he was a suicidal risk. They immediately expressed their concern to their ward personnel. The staff reacted by sending the chairman of the group to meet with the director of the unit. Although steps were taken immediately to locate this patient through the police and family, we were unable to do so before he entered his home and killed himself with a shotgun. Following news of this incident, the patient and staff groups were immediately set in operation to serve as an abreaction channel for their feelings about this incident. This was especially significant to the group to which his girl friend belonged. The group offered immediate support to this patient, dealt with their own fantasies regarding death which helped them to work through some of their own feelings in this area. The impact of this incident was minimal in regard to acting out, and the grief reactions were of short duration.

Epidemics of suicidal attempts are common on an adolescent ward for girls. At one time there were two girls with histrionic personality disorders who were acting out by attempting to cut their wrists. This was immediately picked up in the therapy group, and later the impact of their behavior on the ward was discussed with negative reinforcement by the peer group. The reaction of these girls could be summarized by the statement of one of the 15-year-olds who said "this group just takes all of the fun out of it" in reference to the attempts. Again, here there was action and therapeutic intervention without the need to impose further controls.

For the staff, assignment to such a group provided the opportunity to function very closely together in a number of activities, to distribute roles and functions among themselves according to the needs of the group and the individual, and to provide the context within which mutual training and experiential learning could take place. These staff-patient groups functioned in a variety of ways. Some of the activities were designed to provide the individual patient with intensive interaction with the peer members of his group, independently of staff. Other activities provided equally intensive interaction and communication between patients and staff within a single group. Still other activities were designed to give the individual patient some experience in functioning as a member of the total staff-patient community. Finally, still other activities were designed to give the patient some experience with the larger community outside of the hospital.

Between the peer group, task group and ward government group there were several interrelated tasks, such as setting up their responsibilities regarding some of the daily chores, and organizing activities that would be enjoyable and fun. This group helped some of those complaining of boredom to mobilize and organize activities, by which they found they were able to enjoy them. This involved the budgeting of the trips, scheduling of outside events, contact with the community resources, etc. A resource person from the staff was available to help them find appropriate solutions to their requests. If the peer group had an idea for an activity it was discussed in the task group; then it would be presented to the floor government for discussion. Following this, the Executive Council might take action, if it was necessary, to involve other parts of the total hospital structure, such as securing extra buses or money from volunteers.

The patients in the group were encouraged to hold meetings and discussions together at any time during the day when problems came up with respect to the behavior of one of its members, or in the relationships of the group as a whole to the staff or to the hospital. These "here and now" discussions (Group II), held by the patients with no staff present, provided an opportunity for the development of a group identification and for the exercise of peer pressure upon individual members. Therapeutic solutions of day-to-day problems of group living were possible through the responsibility of the group, rather than through staff intervention.

At times, an adolescent with leadership qualities and psychopathic symptoms may create a group for his own needs. Even here the unit groups could be of extreme help in intervening early. At one point such a patient was organizing a "gang" to defend the "honor" of the unit against outsiders. These outsiders were high school kids who were cutting through the hospital grounds and had made some unkind remarks to one of the girls (the patient's girl friend). The situation was discussed at the peer group level where they attempted to suggest different alternatives. Later there was further exploration and understanding of exploitation and projection. The outcome was that a delegation was formed to discuss the situation with the kids who were passing by, and a liaison staff person was sent to the nearby school to bring this to the attention of the school principal.

It was necessary to arrange for staff members to be available for "consultation" to the peer group. The group at times tended to be rather punitive to some member with deviant behavior. An example of this occurred when one group decided to place a psychotic member in an isolation room for a prolonged period of time with the result that the patient suffered an hallucinatory experience.

At the same time these same groups constituted intensive psychotherapy groups (Group III) held at stated intervals during the week. These intensive therapy group meetings followed more traditional lines, with the exception that all levels of staff assigned to that group were present. There was an opportunity, following each group session, for discussion among the staff about the dynamics of the group, as well as the characteristics and therapeutic needs of individual patients in the group. The opportunity for all levels of staff to develop a psychodynamic orientation toward the patient gave a different meaning to so-called "ward incidents," and enabled staff to deal with these problems in a more therapeutic manner.

The following is an example of how an adolescent acting out in a ward of adult patients in a general hospital brings about the need to impose "controls" and more restriction instead of a therapeutic intervention. Following a frustrating home visit, a 15-year-old borderline psychotic female walked up and down the corridor shouting four-letter words. The reaction from the staff was "we have to stop this" and "what to do," since the other patients were complaining. The nurses asked for more power to control this misbehavior, which they blamed on the physician who was "too permissive" in dealing with this. The discussion at the meeting of staff doctors, where I was "invited" as a "consultant," concerned what to do. The statement made by the patient's physician that he would be more upset if an older patient wandered around his room at midnight was answered by a "that's your problem." A committee had already been established to set guidelines for adolescent patients, but its members were deadlocked in shouting. By this point the dynamics were lost sight of, as was the question of the most therapeutic intervention.

By contrast, a similar incident was handled quite differently with a patient on the unit system. A psychotic 14-year-old boy walked up and down the unit softly striking the shoulders or back of everyone in sight as he passed by, which annoyed all involved. In his psychotherapy group some of the dynamics involved in this compulsive behavior were understood as a need to establish some sort of relationship by touching. After the therapist discussed this in the staff meeting and in the psychotherapy group the patients' awareness of this led them to offer support and friendship to this youngster. The reaction of the group was not to restrain him but to offer more support.

Staff members found that their understanding of the dynamics of action and reaction was not limited to the patients, but involved their own actions, with the possibility of immediate feedback of their involvement in the transference-countertransference of acting out by the staff, who are constantly pressured by the seductiveness of the adolescent. Sometimes the acting out goes the other way, that is, from the staff involved in the treatment of the adolescent toward the outside larger community of the hospital. Reaction from the staff to the hospital administration's statements regarding some increased adolescent acting out on the grounds (exemplified by statements such as "let's build a barbed-wire fence around the center") was one of resentful feelings. At that point, a group of adolescents raided the research lab, setting free a large number of mice and rats, which they distributed around the hospital floors. This was handled with minimal fuss and an almost condoning attitude by the unit staff. Because of the unit structure and function, this lack of reaction was discussed extensively in subsequent meetings. The staff was then able to understand its own emotional involvement with, and subtle stimulation of, this acting out.

The group structure also benefits the staff in many ways. Sometimes understanding has to come in a "hard" way, as one new middle-aged staff member learned in one of the patient groups. When she joined the unit, she had the attitude of "trust-love-care" to all the adolescents without regard to their pathology and without much understanding of her own needs. She left her purse with money in it near an open office door and her money soon disappeared. When the group was called to deal with this incident, one of the patients shouted "sucker." From here on the discussion dealt with seduction of the staff by the adolescents and seduction of the adolescents by the staff. The staff member therefore was able to deal with her own feelings much better now that the "criticism" was coming not only from the authority figure of the director, who had already discussed this with her, but also from the youngsters.

The group also functioned as the instrument whereby duties and responsibilities associated with ward living were discussed and distributed among individual members (Group IV). For example, a group might be assigned certain duties on the ward for a week; the group as a whole would be made responsible for the performances of these duties, and it would be up to the group of patients as a whole to deal with any problems of individual members in the performance of these duties.

Each group of patients elected a chairman, who represented the group in various dealings with other group chairmen and staff, and who also led the patient discussion sessions or "Government" (Group V). This structure encouraged individual responsibility and provided the individual patient with social recognition and increased self-esteem. As for the benefits of this group, we are in accord with Jones (1953) "that all this can have a socializing value, whatever the dynamics may be . . ." It also provided the patient in the group with a buffer or intermediary through which he could make his needs known to the staff, with staff present who had no vote.

The representatives of these groups would meet together by themselves (Group VI) in the so-called "Patient Executive Council" to discuss various kinds of problems of their groups and decide what to present to the staff as a total group problem. They had an opportunity to meet with staff representatives at least once a week or on an emergency basis. They could review problems of ward functioning, plan for group activities and voice dissatisfaction and complaints which they felt were being experienced by their groups. This information could then be communicated by the staff representatives to all staff members at a general staff conference. The patient representatives communicated back to their groups the results of their discussions with the staff, and had the responsibility of guiding group discussions within their own groups, as well as enlisting the cooperation of members in group tasks and group activities. These leaders were elected by their group and the leadership was rotated every month. Another task of this council was to present requests for activities or grievances involving aspects beyond the unit's administration, for which they met regularly with the unit director. An example of this was the wish to change "curfew" hours that were set up by the hospital administration. When necessary, they were able to present their complaints directly to the hospital superintendent. This allowed for the exercise of leadership and developing feelings of acceptance and channeled their feelings in a constructive way in dealing with the external reality of the rest of the community.

Attempts were made to establish similar groups with parents but this proved to be quite difficult and only two groups were formed that followed more traditional counseling lines (Group VII). This failure was possibly related to the social background of our population, e.g., high incidence of broken or disorganized homes, and realities, such as lack of transportation, etc. At times these attempts to include the parents were a complete failure, e.g., when the patients organized a ceremony related to their Scout activities, only one mother and one grandmother were present. Slightly more success ensued when other activities, such as parties, were organized.

In brief, the individual patient was provided with the opportunity for intensive interaction and communication within his own peer group or with other peers in the community; he could communicate with staff directly within his group or on an individual basis, or through his representatives. Also, he could communicate on a more intimate level within the therapy group, or with the entire ward community at ward meetings.

In order to maintain coordination and communication among all staff, a series of conferences was instituted, which enabled every staff member to have direct interaction and communication with every other staff member at least once during the week (Group I). The general staff meeting held once weekly consisted of all staff working with patients, including physicians, occupational therapists, educators, ward personnel, psychologists, and social workers assigned to the ward. The planning of the total program of therapy for the individual patient was based on these discussions. In addition to this, conferences were held once weekly by the psychiatrist director with the nursing staff in which medical and administrative problems could be reviewed in detail. This meeting was especially important, since it included personnel from all three shifts and formed the basic point of communication between the day and evening/night shifts. In addition to this, social workers, psychologists, psychiatric residents, and the director himself all made themselves available for consultation with individual members of the ward staff with respect to any kind of problem which that staff member might wish to discuss.

We were also concerned with the problem of helping the adolescent to reestablish some type of constructive activity within the community. Our experience indicated that the typical adolescent who is hospitalized feels a deep sense of shame, loss of self-esteem and feelings of rejection. These attitudes, whether primarily projections or reality, handicap him in his attempts to reintegrate himself into the community. It was therefore important to provide him with social experiences with individuals and organizations from the community, in order that these attitudes might be modified. For this reason we instituted a program of activities in which the adolescent patients were either involved in some common activity with a community organization outside of the hospital, or where individuals and organizations from the community participated in some aspect of their hospital activities within the hospital grounds. Included here were Scout activities, volunteer work, camping, etc. This program was made possible through the very active volunteer program already existing in the hospital. We were seriously hampered in this program by hospital regulations covering hospital-community activities, which prohibited nursing personnel from participating fully in these activities.

We would like to point out that a residential setting is almost a "marathon" grouping with twenty-four hours of group interaction for weeks or months. The above organization offers the necessary structure for positive interaction and growth of these groups. We feel Szurek's (1971) comment merits repetition: "The need to validate his own reactions, feelings, thoughts with another undergoing similar experience appears insatiable."

SUMMARY

The admission of increasing numbers of adolescents from 12 to 17 years of age created a therapeutic problem at this hospital. Unique therapeutic requirements of this patient group necessitated the establishment of a program markedly different from what had existed previously for an adult psychotic population. An analysis of the procedures which existed in the hospital led us to recognize a number of deficiencies in organization and procedures which we felt would seriously handicap any treatment program with adolescents. For this reason, we developed a unit characterized by several important differences.

First, the organizational structure which we established was designed to develop a task-oriented treatment team. Secondly, the establishment of multi-functional groups was designed to (a) fulfill the therapeutic needs of the patients with respect to individual problems and problems of group living, (b) facilitate the distribution of skills and competence among the staff through close collaborative participation in group activities, and (c) facilitate the intercommunication and establishment of flexible staff roles which were essential to the operation of such a unit.

A major change is required to provide a large degree of autonomy for such a unit, so that therapeutic procedures appropriate to the needs of the adolescent patient can be developed. Such units require the development of a high degree of cohesiveness and intercommunication among staff, and intensive training which can enable the staff to function in a variety of therapeutic roles. These requirements involve an initial period of learning experiences in new modes of functioning. It is expected that during the first six months of operation such a unit will go through many internal crises, as well as conflicts vis-à-vis the rest of the hospital. The working through of problems of staff role relationships, the experimentation with different organizational structures, and the learning required to function effectively in new roles are part of the development of a treatment milieu. Finally, on both theoretical and practical grounds, the development of staff-patient "reference groups" within the unit would seem to provide the most effective structure around which the entire treatment program can be oriented and to provide maximum development of staff potentials.

One of our hopes—that this system would maintain the personnel and reduce the turnover—was achieved. Although we do not have actual figures to compare, we can say that within the period of functioning of the system, the personnel turnover was low. Even with the unavoidable changes of the staff assigned for training, the groups were able to maintain the structure that minimized the impact of these changes, with a more even flow of the treatment process.

We think that this type of organization of interlocking groups, which facilitates communication and negotiable transaction among staff, can be of benefit to many residential centers, whether short-term or long-term, and is especially valuable for large institutions.

REFERENCES

AUERSWALD, E. (1969). Changing concepts and changing models of residential treatment. In *Adolescence: Psychosocial Perspectives*. G. Caplan and S. Lebovici, eds. New York: Basic Books.

DEUTSCH, H. (1967). *Selected Problems of Adolescence.* Monograph Series of the Psychoanalytic Study of the Child. New York: International Universities Press.

FREUD, A. (1969). Adolescence as a developmental disturbance. In *Adolescence: Psychosocial Perspectives.* G. Caplan and S. Lebovici, eds. New York: Basic Books.

HENRY, J. (1957). Types of institutional structure. *Psychiatry,* 20:47-60.

JONES, M. (1953). *The Therapeutic Community.* New York: Basic Books.

KAHNE, M. J. (1959). Bureaucratic structure and impersonal experience in mental hospitals. *Psychiatry,* 12:363-375.

KRAFT, I. A. (1971). Child and adolescent group psychotherapy. In *Comprehensive Group Therapy.* I. Kaplan and B. Sadock, eds. Baltimore: Williams & Wilkins Co.

SZUREK, S. A. (1971). The needs of adolescents for emotional health. In *Modern Perspectives in Adolescent Psychiatry.* J. Howells, ed. New York: Brunner/Mazel.

6

The Impact of Group Experiences on Adolescent Development

ROGER L. SHAPIRO, M.D., JOHN ZINNER, M.D.,
DAVID A. BERKOWITZ, M.D., *and*
EDWARD R. SHAPIRO, M.D.

Experiences of adolescents in family and group situations are central determinants of their evolving identity (Erikson, 1956, Shapiro, 1963). Over the past decade, our research at the National Institute of Mental Health on adolescent personality formation has included study of both family and group relations of healthy and disturbed adolescents. Our aim has been to specify types of transactions within the family and the group which contribute to healthy or disturbed personality development and functioning in the adolescent. We have reported findings regarding family determinants of adolescent personality formation in a number of publications (Berkowitz et al., 1973; Shapiro, E. et al., in press; Shapiro, R., 1967, 1968, 1969; Shapiro, R. and Zinner, in press; Zinner and Shapiro, R., 1974; Zinner and Shapiro, E., 1974).

In this paper we shall consider some aspects of the adolescent's experiences in groups and social institutions which have consequences for his evolving ego identity. Specifically, from the data of our group work with adolescents, we shall consider three interrelated themes which have impact upon identity formation: the adolescent's definition of himself in the group and the group's delineation of him, the adolescent's defensive use of the group, and the adolescent's experience with and reaction to authority.

This paper comes from work done in association with Carmen Amoros-Cabrera, M.A., Doris Droke, and Gay Grover, R.N.

The core of Erikson's discussion of identity formation is its integration of psychosocial experience with psychological epigenesis (Erikson, 1950, 1956, 1962). During adolescence, the ego's task of achieving continuity and integration in self-definition is particularly acute because of new maturation both in the ego and in the drives (Blos, 1962; Freud, 1936; Inhelder and Piaget, 1958). Related to this maturation, the adolescent experiences rapidly changing social definitions of himself. The psychological growth of the adolescent leads to an extensive reorganization of the personality structure of childhood (Freud, 1958; Jacobson, 1964). This is shaped not only by the nature of internalizations of childhood experience, but also by the adolescent's current experiences in his family, in groups, and in institutions in society. In these current psychosocial situations, the adolescent must develop an integration of new experiences with important past experiences in order to establish a coherent sense of identity.

We investigate three interrelated aspects of the adolescent's group experience significant for identity formation. First is the delineation of the individual adolescent by the group and the relation of this to his definition of himself. By "delineation" we mean the group's communication to the adolescent of perceptions of him and attitudes toward him (Shapiro, 1967). Delineations may either be explicitly spoken or implicitly expressed in group members' behavior toward the adolescent. Group delineations have a powerful impact on the individual adolescent: their characteristics determine the role he is assigned by the group.

A second and related aspect of group experience involves the defensive uses the adolescent makes of the group. When the group is used defensively, we frequently see transactions between group members based upon a dynamic of projective identification (Zinner and Shapiro, R., 1974). This phenomenon is observed in behaviors in which the individual adolescent projects conflictful aspects of himself into other group members with whom he then identifies. In this way, he need not suffer the anxiety of taking responsibility for these characteristics in himself with, however, important consequences for his own personality functioning and evolving identity. He may then continue to disown significant components of his impulse life or conscience, rather than achieving internalization and integration of these needs and controls into a stable ego identity during adolescence.

A third aspect of the adolescent's group experience important to our study is his changing relationship to people in authority. As he moves from his family to experiences in groups and social institutions, personality reorganization in the adolescent requires both an integration of new delineations of him by authority figures and modification of his projections into them. In our work with families of healthy adolescents we have observed characteristics of parental behavior which support central tasks of adolescent development: individuation, separation, and the finding of new objects. In families with seriously disturbed adolescents, we observe characteristics of parental behavior and infer unconscious assumptions in the family as a group which do not support, but rather militate against accomplishment of the developmental tasks of adolescence (Berkowitz et al., 1973; Shapiro, E. et al., in press; Shapiro, R. and Zinner, in press; Zinner and Shapiro, R., 1974).

Family experiences have important consequences for the adolescent's relationships to authority figures in groups outside of his family. They affect his capacity to use that leadership which promotes group behavior, learning and work in the adolescent, and which utilizes his new potentialities and develops his competence. The quality of his relationships with his parents orients the adolescent's relationship to new authority figures into whom he projects attitudes determined by past relationships which may either promote or interfere with his capacity to work in new group situations.

Important continuities exist between the individual's experience in his family (his first group), and his subsequent behavior in groups. We consider these continuities in the areas of response to new delineations, defensive use of the group, and fundamental attitudes toward authority. The interplay between family experience and group experience and the adolescent's capacity to integrate these experiences parallels the important libidinal move of the adolescent from his primary objects, his parents, to new libidinal objects in his own age group. This shift is generally conceptualized in dyadic (pre-oedipal) or triadic (oedipal) terms. In this paper we suggest another level of conceptualization of adolescent behavior and experience, that of his experience in groups which derives from family experience and shapes identity formation.

THEORETICAL BACKGROUND

Our theory of family organization, as well as our orientation to groups, derive from the small group theory of Bion (1961). We characterize families as functioning on two levels with regard to the family's task of promoting the development of children (Shapiro, R. and Zinner, in press). The first level of family functioning consists of behavior which supports and facilitates the child's and adolescent's accomplishment of phase-appropriate developmental tasks. From the point of view of adolescent development, we define the task of the family as the promotion of relative ego autonomy and individuation in the adolescent leading to identity consolidation and psychological separation from his parents. Family behavior in support of this task is regulated by the reality principle and mediated primarily through secondary process thinking.

At a second level of functioning of the family as a group, the level of unconscious assumptions, family behavior is determined by shared unconscious fantasies mobilized more by instinctual needs or defensive requirements within the family than by realistic developmental considerations. Family functioning determined by unconscious assumptions may be mobilized when behavior appropriate to a new phase of development is initiated. Anxiety, regressive and defensive behaviors, disturbances in communication, and interference in the family's reality functioning ensue, resulting in serious failures in family task performance with regard to the development of the child or adolescent.

Correspondingly, in the group experience of adolescents, work tasks are interfered with by the mobilization of unconscious assumptions. If, in his group experience, the adolescent avoids reality tasks and uses the group defensively without taking responsibility for his feelings and behavior, he will have difficulty in work groups, with serious consequences for his developing skills and competence. Bion's theory helps us elucidate states in groups in which there is a movement away from reality functioning and work, and to consider the role the adolescent is taking in relation to basic assumption leadership and the maintenance of the basic assumption life of the group. The unconscious assumptions which govern family life are often highly specific unconscious fantasies determined by the personality organization of the parents and their transactions with developing children and adolescents over time. In contrast, the basic assumption fantasies of groups occur without a long developmental history and reflect powerful general unconscious themes in group psychology.

In Bion's (1961) conceptualization, groups are defined by the task they are gathered to perform, and they function on two levels which may or may not complement one another (Bion, 1961; Rioch, 1970; Turquet, 1971). Group behavior on the first level is referred to as work group functioning. It is task-oriented and guided primarily by the reality principle and secondary process thinking. Bion observes that much behavior in groups appears to have some other motivation than work. This behavior suggests another level of group functioning in which there is an unconscious assumption on the part of the members that the group is gathered for a quite different purpose than the realistic accomplishment of the work task. Bion postulates unconscious mechanisms in group members which are mobilized in group interrelationships and which result in behavior unconcerned with the considerations of reality such as task implementation, logical thinking, and time. He designates as basic assumptions those states in groups where behavior appears to be determined by wishful and nonrational unconscious considerations. In such states a group appears to be dominated and often united by covert assumptions based on unconscious fantasies in relation to authority and leadership.

Bion outlines three general categories of basic assumptions which he frequently sees dominating the behavior of groups. One is the unconscious assumption that the group exists for satisfaction of dependency needs and wishes (basic assumption dependency); another is the assumption that the group exists to promote aggression toward or to provide the means of flight from reality issues and tasks (basic assumption fight-flight); the third is an assumption of hope and an atmosphere of expectation which is unrelated to reality considerations and is frequently seen in relation to pairing behavior in the group (basic assumption pairing).

The basic assumption mode of group behavior, then, is formulated from behavior which implies covert and often unconscious assumptions in group members about the purpose for which the group is gathered. These assumptions, which have little to do with considerations of reality, have powerful unconscious determinants and are conceptualized as expressions of shared unconscious fantasies in group members.

The adolescent's experiences in school, in work, and in other social institutions define crucial components of his ego identity. He may seek group experiences in which basic assumption life predominates and in which the leadership he takes or relates to is basic assumption leadership. His avoidance of reality tasks in groups may generate sufficient difficulty in work groups to result in school and work failure with serious consequences for his evolving sense of identity. Identity confusion, which has its origin in the dynamics of family relationships, is then aggravated by the adolescent's group experiences. However, the adolescent's development will be facilitated if, in his group experiences, he is able to join the work leadership of his groups and find a constructive relationship with individuals in authority in his institutions. Instead of using the groups defensively, he will then be able to take increasing responsibility in work groups and will develop skills and new competence. His group experiences will contribute to the increasing ego autonomy and individuation essential for healthy identity consolidation.

CLINICAL SETTING

Our treatment program for adolescents who are seriously disturbed takes recognition of the importance of their group experience through therapeutic work with the adolescents in groups, in addition to family treatment and individual psychotherapy. In our residential treatment program we have worked with over 50 adolescents, ages 14-21, and their families. The adolescents all manifest severe identity confusion with diagnoses ranging from borderline disorders to severe character disorders to neurotic disorders.

Therapeutic modalities include both individual psychotherapy for the adolescent, conjoint family therapy, and study of the hospital group in which the adolescent lives and works. The program combines three hours per week of individual psychotherapy for the adolescent with a weekly one-hour conjoint family therapy session, one hour per week of marital therapy for the parents, a weekly multiple family meeting, and three patient-staff meetings per week, including one which is a study group examining peer relations and authority relations on the psychiatric unit. In addition, the patients meet weekly themselves as a group to make recommendations for unit government. The program is designed to allow us to consider the psychological maturation of the individual adolescent in relation to his experiences within his family, within his peer group, and within the social institution of which he is a part.

In the patient-staff meetings the rules which regulate life on the unit are evolved, issues concerning implementation of the school and work program are discussed, activities away from the clinical center are decided upon, and community passes and privileges are requested and discussed by the group. Efforts are made to examine the responsibility each patient is taking for therapy, school, work, and behavior in the hospital and outside community. In order to study and modify the dynamics of these meetings, we hold another meeting each week, a one-hour unit study group. This is an intergroup meeting consisting of all of the patients, the chief psychiatric nurse representing the nursing staff, the unit psychiatric administrator representing the individual and family therapists, and the clinical director representing the research project chiefs and senior psychiatric staff. The task of this meeting is defined as study of peer relations and authority relations in the group life of the psychiatric unit. It is explicit that this is not a decision-making meeting, but one in which the dynamics of roles and role relationships are studied, including the nature of attitudes toward those in authority roles.

The work of the unit study group is the examination of roles individuals are put into or take in the hospital group in which they live and work. In this work, we focus upon transactions within the group in which the adolescent is delineated by the group, or defines himself, in relation to peers or to authority. We attend in particular to changes in these delineations and self-definitions in the group setting, and the dynamics of change over time. This is the focus of our interpretive work.

A whole range of issues of group life in the hospital is discussed in this group. We study the relationships between the adolescents and staff members in authority roles with attention to both the real and the fantasied characteristics of these relationships. The task of the group is a difficult one, and the adolescents frequently resist joining the leadership which staff members provide. The adolescents often attempt to change the work of the group and take leadership to move the group in the direction of basic assumption life. Consistent interpretive work on the part of the staff is required to clarify the dynamics of struggle between work and basic assumption leadership and to promote the joining by the adolescents in a therapeutic work task of self-observation and study. The adolescents may then take increasing responsibility for their own behavior in the group, work more freely in the area of self-definition, and decrease their defensive projection into the group of both impulses and dictates of conscience which they disown in themselves. Through examining their frequent abdications of responsibility in response to the authority of staff members, they develop an increasing sense of their responsibility for their own behavior and for the roles they take on the hospital unit.

CLINICAL MATERIAL: SELF-DEFINITION, DELINEATION AND AUTHORITY RELATIONS

The following excerpt from a Unit Study Group meeting contains a discussion of patient silence, apathy, and withdrawal from the task of the group. Dr. S (the clinical director) delineates the patients as feeling like the "low man on the totem pole," and, in consequence, the patients are surrendering their personal authority and competence to work in the group. The patients respond with several different self-definitions. Bruce is mobilized into work leadership and defines the authority he has to understand himself as well as his anger at being delineated by others. Carol defines herself as too preoccupied with her own self and her individual boundaries to work in the group. Arnold defines his own and the group's covert efforts to engage basic assumption leaders in the areas of both dependency and fight-flight.

EXCERPT

Dr. S: One consequence I was thinking of is that if less talk has to do with having less authority, then the patients feel low man on the totem pole.

Bruce: Yeah, but you know, the way I see it is that you cats can tell us things forever, you know, but it wouldn't do any good, like, 'cause each person is an individual and you can't—like if you're going to help somebody with their problems or something you're going to have to know that individual pretty well, and, like, you can't just come and tell people what's happening, they have to tell *you*, you know. If they don't tell you then you really can't do a very effective job. So you can sit and talk forever and it's not gonna do any good. And you can tell 'em where it's at. It might even *be* that way . . . but you really don't *know* where they're at 'cause they won't talk to you.

Dr. S: I couldn't agree more!

Bruce: Well . . . that's where it's at, I think. . . .

Dr. R: It's not clear why you want to, for instance, leave me as unit administrator not knowing where you're at, so that it makes the administration not accurate, sort of imposed.

Bruce: Well, I don't *know*. I just think, *you* might feel it starts off like I'm leaving you there, but *I* feel like it starts off like you're imposing on *me*. You know what I mean?

Dr. R: So it's a debatable question as to who started imposing on whom, and there's a battle going on . . . ?

Bruce: [*interrupting*] It really doesn't matter. I don't see any battle, really . . . you know. . . .

Dr. R: Sounds like it.

Bruce: [*Snickers*]

Dr. S: I think it's clarifying. I have a lot of feeling of people feeling imposed on. But you're also saying something about your knowing best of all where it's at for you.

Bruce: That's right.

Dr. S: And that's true for everyone in this room.

Bruce: [*Low voice*] That's right.

Dr. R: You know, I think that Fred was empathic with the position he felt me to be in, at least he could see that I was sitting alone. Now it's almost as if pointing that out and making an effort seems to have worn him out. Takes a lot of work. Carol points out everybody's alone to some degree. Sounds like she felt very alone. Yet to work on what that's about— maybe it's about being with people who tend to talk too much so you feel like they're imposing. It takes more effort than it seems to be worth.

Carol: [*Pause*] Well, I think each person in here was—attempting to— bound their own territory, you know . . . create—their own world, their own boundaries.

Dr. R: How do you go about doing that, Carol?

Carol: What?

Dr. R: Sorting out—your place.

Carol: I haven't been involved in that here. . . .

Dr. R: You haven't at all? . . . sounds like you've been thinking about it.

Carol: Well, I was—thinking more in terms of my own place, not— with other people, but with myself. Your way—of forming boundaries is talking and—getting everything in form, all your actions and interactions, so—

Dr. S: [*Pause*] Are you saying that's not *your* way?

Carol: I'm just saying that it's one way.

Arnold: One thing I have noticed about this meeting is that it seems to be a rather odd relationship here between staff and patients in that they do interact but they never seem to work quite properly. It never seems to get anywhere, and I was wondering why. I just was reading *The Autobiography of Malcolm X*. You know, the more you read, the more you get turned on to the fact that the audiences in certain parts of the countries that Malcolm X was visiting were actually putting on little vignettes. They were acting. So Malcolm X would be struck by this, just as Nixon was struck by that girl who was holding up the sign some place in Ohio. There is a definite interrelationship between the actor or the audience, and uh—the leader. Like they are two parts of the whole.

Dr. S: [*Pause*] One could say that your model of Malcolm X and the countries he visited, or even President Nixon for that matter and the girl he saw saying "Bring us together," that there is something going on in this room similar to that.

Arnold: Similar, yeah, but it seems to be descending, spiraling downwards as opposed to the opposite, spiraling upwards.

Dr. S: I think it's felt so much as a slap in the face; for instance, I called Bruce the group artist and—he— winced as if I'd struck him and insulted him.

Bruce: I don't want to be the group artist.

Dr. S: I was saying what my perception was of you. You didn't say that you didn't want to be that or what you did want to be or anything. You winced and looked angry.

Bruce: Yeah, man, you know, you can just go on saying whatever you want to say, it's fine.

Dr. S: I don't say whatever I want to say.

Bruce: Maybe you should.

Dr. S: Maybe I should? No, I try to think about what I say. There is a job we are trying to do here. Some things I think don't have anything to do with that and I wouldn't say them.

Arnold: Must we have such areas of controversy. There probably could be things we could talk about going on outside of the unit.

Dr. S: Outside of the unit.

Arnold: Of course, it's probably too irrelevant to what's happening. I think it's a better idea than sitting around here sighing and being afraid to talk.

Dr. R: It sounds like you're on to the drama going on right in here.

Arnold: How so?

Dr. R: Malcolm X comes to mind. . . .

Arnold: Well, it's just, just that I happened to be reading it. He thought that the audience was reacting strictly to him. He didn't realize that the audience, people who were watching him, were trying to impress something upon his mind also. By the way the audience as a whole was reacting. He never considered this, how his policies were changed by the people he talked to. You know, the reception he got influenced his mind and his actions.

In this excerpt Bruce is taking new initiative in transactions with authority figures through stating the patient's responsibility for defining the boundaries of their individuality. They are the authorities on who they are and what their problems are. There is recognition that unless they let staff authority figures know how they think and feel, the staff is unable to do its job. However, anger over feelings of being controlled and imposed upon continues to deflect his work leadership into the direction of fight. Carol contributes to the understanding of patient anonymity. She says she is too preoccupied with establishing her individual boundaries to be able to deal with the group at all at this time.

Arnold makes a perceptive statement about the group's communication to leaders. He says leaders can tell from the way the group is behaving what the group needs and wants, and he describes the group's power to influence the leaders and to get something from them. The group's communications of feelings of need and wishes for cohesion may take precedence over the work of the group. Arnold is also disturbed by Bruce's fight with Dr. S and Dr. R and wants to lead the group away from internal areas of controversy. He protests the doctors' efforts to focus on the group task of study and self-definition. He implies that the patients, through their messages that they are helpless and must be cared for, want to use the group for a different task than understanding their group life.

The group is dominated by covert assumptions of dependency upon the professional staff members and of fight-flight. These are pervasive dynamics to which the patients relate in a variety of ways. They appear to feel needful, helpless, and highly vulnerable to authority figures. They perceive authority as extremely coercive and want to fight it. Arnold is describing the power of the group members to affect work leaders in his Malcolm X metaphor. In this meeting wishes for care from authority figures are expressed through group members acting helpless and fearful, and there is anger in the meeting both over feelings of vulnerability and because of frustrated dependency. The fight is being expressed primarily by Bruce. Arnold's statement that Malcolm X didn't consider how his policies were changed by the people he talked to defines what is happening to work leadership in this meeting in which patients repeatedly attempt to evoke from the staff a basic assumption leadership of dependency and take leadership themselves in fight-flight. This takes precedence over self-definition and definition of the experience of the group which is the work task of the group.

How do we accomplish work in this group situation with the powerful basic assumption dynamics which exist in it? Work is promoted through our position that the patients are responsible for their participation and contribution in the group as they are responsible for their behavior in the hospital. Their participation in our program is voluntary and represents a choice which they have made for which they are responsible. The patients often want to deny this responsibility and to locate it within their parents or the staff. They often want to insist upon their helplessness and their inability to behave responsibly. At the same time they express hatred toward the professional staff for exercising control over them. They want to deny that they themselves have any role in relinquishing their own controls and their own responsibility.

CLINICAL MATERIAL: THE USE OF GROUP EXPERIENCES
FOR DEFENSIVE PURPOSES; EXTERNALIZATION OF
RESPONSIBILITY AND OF CONFLICT

In order to promote the goal of the patient group taking responsibility for its behavior and for the behavior of individual members, we encouraged the patients to meet weekly without staff present to review patient behavior and to make recommendations for patient privileges. These became important discussions, the reports of which were highly useful, for the patients frequently knew more about what was going on among their peers than the staff did and often empathically understood the significance of the behavior of their peers. This group meeting, however, went counter to the basic assumption dependency functioning of the patient group, which wanted the continued exercise of authority by the staff. Initially, despite its charge, the patient group, meeting alone, sought to externalize responsibility onto the staff and felt abandoned when the nurturance of staff direction was not forthcoming. This is indicated poignantly by the verbatim patient summary of such a meeting:

> Notes were taken by Carol last week and she did not write down many details about any discussion that took place. Last week's meeting was more than the notes revealed. There is a need for more precise, detailed notes because that is really what the staff has to go on in rounds. There is a lot of silence in today's meeting. People are like ten "islands," which is descriptive of the past meetings. People are looking at doing two things at one time—concern for one's self and concern for others. Staff absence in this meeting is felt. The feeling is that if staff leads a meeting it is easier. Patients are each trying to lead or each taking a share in the responsibility.

The bereft, uncohesive quality of the group emerges starkly in this record. A corollary to the dependency on staff is the obvious loss of skills of the patients marked by the lack of detail in the notes and the preponderance of silence.

With continued working in group meetings on the dynamics of basic assumption dependency, the patients gradually demonstrated increasing willingness to take responsibility. Again, quoting from notes of a later meeting of the patient group:

> Patients feel that they should take a part in responsibility on a trip. If some patient is irresponsible, other patients should take the re-

sponsibility. Patients don't want to give one or two patients power to turn the whole trip back. If something happens, there should be a meeting upon return to determine actions to be taken on certain patients.

As patients began to take leadership in the group, we observed a tendency to identify with the aggressor, that is, with the fantasied most primitive and harsh aspects of the staff. The group would mete out severe restrictions on individual members for mild infractions, with group members projecting their own unintegrated impulses into that member as *the* wrongdoer, while maintaining an illusion that they were free of such impulses and desires themselves. Such a group dynamic did not further the important task of superego reorganization in the patients leading to more harmonious internal integration of drive and prohibition. It was effective in controlling acting out among patients, but from the individual's perspective the prohibitions remained externalized. Furthermore, the projection of the group's shared conflicts into one member spared the rest of the patients the anxiety of experiencing conflict within themselves. In the following patient meeting notes, the group is wrestling with such an issue:

> Arnold talked about his mother moving back in the house, mainly because of his therapist saying that the family would be put out of the program if she didn't. People expressed some feelings and thoughts they had concerning their own parents and separation. But for the most part, people seem very afraid to speak on this subject and talk in generalities and seem to think more about separation of parents in other families than their own. Or else expressed thoughts about parents separating in the past. Arnold was very pissed off because he thought that people were leaving the subject of separation with him and not looking at their own parents and separation. Fantasies were expressed about parents splitting up and which parent they would live with.

Here Arnold has acted as a work leader by directing the group back to the problem of separation as a shared fear, and the group responds with group members internalizing their own concerns, rather than projecting them and vicariously experiencing those of Arnold. He reversed a process of externalization in the group, thus allowing group members to work intrapsychically on shared conflicts and anxieties about the stability of their parents' marriages. Borderline adolescents characteristically use projective and splitting defenses and are particularly prone to use the group for externalization of conflict through projection. It is a task of work leadership to counter this defensive use of the group, and to redirect group members towards processes of internalization and integration of conflictful feelings and issues.

Our focus upon defensive uses the adolescents make of the group on the ward has been central to the work of the unit study group. It has been the means of exploring major psychological issues of its component members and provides an important resource for the adolescent's psychological development. Our patients, at least in the early stages of hospitalization, perceive the unit study group in the image of their nuclear family relationships. A patient is inclined to promote acting out in his peers as a vicarious way of recreating the very conflicts with family which beset him and which brought him into the hospital.

In the following excerpts, taken from a meeting of the unit study group, we can see the transformation in one patient, Bob, of conflict which initially is externalized in the group meeting. Work during the session leads to internalization of the conflict and contributes to Bob's insight into his own dilemma. This is accomplished through the work leadership both of his peers and the staff members who participate in the meeting.

Bob has been covertly encouraging another patient, Ruth, to run away. Ruth has been contemplating this action because her old therapist is leaving and she is angry and fearful about her transition to a new one. Other members of the patient group are taking Bob to task in the meeting for his secretive talks with Ruth and his unwillingness to urge her to remain. They claim that Ruth and Bob have isolated themselves from the rest of the patient group and are treating it with contempt. Two subgroups are identified, the "good guys," who are most of the patients, and the "bad guys," consisting of Ruth, Bob, and Carol. Bob justifies this split in the following comment:

> I was just thinking about the relationships one-to-one versus relationships one-to-the-group. And thinking that the one-to-one relationship I have with Ruth, I don't see where she's avoiding *me* or anything. I feel like, you know, I can see where there isn't much of a relationship with Ruth and the group. But with Ruth and me as an individual, I think it's pretty good, and I can talk to her. This morning I was talking to Ruth and Carol for quite awhile. It wasn't just one-to-one this morning. It was Ruth and Carol and me and we were talking about things. I think we share some feelings about, well, Ruth's feelings about maybe her relationship with the group and my relationship with the group. Because a lot of times I don't see the group as being much of a group. And I can have more mean-

ingful relationships with people on a one-to-one basis if I want it to come about.

Further investigation by the group encourages Bob to expand upon his feeling of being set off from the rest of the group. Specifically, he begins to take some responsibility for his own anger:

> I don't know how to describe the inpatient group, and it couldn't really be called a group. You know, that's why I'm thinking it was a "patient body." And somehow the—visualizing the patient body, kind of, arms and legs and whatever—and I was trying to think of who's going to be the head of that. It's missing certain parts. Important parts. And it's split. The one thing, though, that kind of makes me turn away sometimes is Joan [a nurse], her being a staff member and all the talk she's been doing lately. I think that's partially it, because it seems like in some ways she's like the ringleader of a group that's been bothering me somehow. It seems too much like she's trying to be a guide somehow and when I'm talking with someone like that that's really trying to put themselves in a position to guide me, I can't really do much work. Unless it's just kind of one-to-one, and I'm feeling like an equal somehow. And seen that way. Because she starts really overdoing it, I think. Trying to play therapist a lot of times, and she comes up with an interpretation and throws it on the floor, you know, and says, "That's the way it is." And it's more that than throwing it on the floor and saying, "This is my idea and let's hear some other ideas." It seems to me that she tries to make a fact out of her own ideas. It seems like my own ideas aren't that much my ideas anymore because it's going through the main interpreter or something. You know, it is kind of put together and then thrown out and that's the way it is.

Here Bob is dealing in a patient-staff meeting with important transference issues. He visualizes the group as a body needing a head. Although he cannot trust his own or other patients' leadership, he also has difficulty using the leadership of the staff. His problems with Nurse Joan derive from serious difficulties with his mother, upon whom he is extremely dependent and of whom he feels terrified. Mother is an overbearing, tempestuous, intrusive woman who imposes her concept of reality on Bob. Mother is the "main interpreter" Bob is referring to who makes Bob "feel like my own ideas aren't that much my ideas anymore."

With continued encouragement Bob elaborates on more sources of his anger against the staff and peer group. He acknowledges his difficulty expressing anger directly and recognizes how he encourages the more emotive Ruth to do it for him:

You know, I think Ruth's been the spokesman for me a couple of times before. Maybe she's been spokesman for herself, but some of the things she's described about herself describe me also. I was thinking about last week and all this business going on with Sharon (another patient) doing all the drugs and everything. I was really kind of pissed off at Sharon but not saying anything about it last week because I didn't want to stir up a great big fight and defensive battle with you [Sharon] by bringing it up because you'd get all defensive and saying "this isn't so." So I didn't say it 'til today. And it was something that I was thinking about. I talked to Ruth about it when Ruth was sitting next to me and you came through a couple of times. I felt kind of angry and then I felt somehow Ruth and I shared the same feelings about you. But I didn't speak about them. It seems like Ruth said more about them than I did. And I allowed her to do that. And I just didn't want to get in a hassle myself. And just kind of let things be, or just kind of let Ruth do the talking.

Within this interaction one can see a shift in Bob's use of the group from a position of defense to a progressive re-internalization of conflict. At the outset he was encouraging the angry acting out of a peer with no awareness of the relation of this behavior to his own anger at staff members, particularly the nurse Joan and at the patient group. By the end of the meeting he was acknowledging his own feelings with awareness of his vicarious exploitation of his fellow patient Ruth and of his fear of his own hostility. This transition did not occur spontaneously. It required a firm commitment to the work task by the peer group and participating staff. This involved a group desire to keep Ruth in treatment, a willingness to see Ruth's potential departure as a product of transactions occurring within the group as well as a wish to understand and help those who were encouraging her to leave. Each of these tasks could have been undermined by basic assumption leadership and group behavior determined by shared unconscious motivations to fight the staff and its authority through encouraging Ruth to take flight.

This episode underscores our major theme. Group experience can be supportive of the progressive development of the adolescent's capacities to think and to work. Or in his group experience the adolescent may avoid reality tasks and use the group defensively without taking responsibility for his feelings and behavior, with serious consequences for his development. Group experiences which encourage processes of internalization within component members rather than defensive splitting, externalization, and projection contribute to ego integration and promote psychological growth.

The patients tend to repeat in the unit study group roles they have taken and are taking in their families. The ongoing task of the group is to work to understand and to modify stereotyped and defensive role behavior which is manifested in the self definitions of the individual adolescent and maintained by group delineations. The adolescent becomes aware of new possibilities for behavior in relation to peers and authority figures in a social organization away from his family. He develops the support and freedom to attempt new behavior. In this way his group experience helps him resume the task, interrupted in the period of identity confusion, of learning and integrating appropriate, mature, and responsible social roles.

SUMMARY

In summary, we have argued that during adolescence there is a continuity between experiences in the family and consequent experiences in groups and social institutions which parallels the libidinal move of the adolescent from his primary objects within the family to new libidinal objects. This latter shift is generally conceptualized in dyadic (pre-oedipal) or triadic (oedipal) terms. In this paper we suggest another level of conceptualization of adolescent behavior and experience, that of his experiences in groups, which derives from his family experience and affects identity formation. We have proposed a conceptualization of family and group experiences which highlights their continuity based upon the small group theory of Bion. Within this framework we have discussed clinical examples from structured groups in our treatment program to illustrate three aspects of the adolescent group experience related to his evolving ego identity. These are the adolescent's definition of himself and the group delineations of him, the adolescent's defensive use of the group and the adolescent's reaction to authority. These themes, which originate in the family, are greatly elaborated in the adolescent's life in groups and social institutions, and further shape his identity.

REFERENCES

BERKOWITZ, D., SHAPIRO, R., ZINNER, J., SHAPIRO, E. (In press). Family contributions to narcissistic disturances in adolescents. *Int. Rev. Psychoanalysis.*

BION, W. R. (1961). *Experience in Groups.* London: Tavistock Publications.

BLOS, P. (1962). *On Adolescence: A Psychoanalytic Interpretation.* New York: The Free Press of Glencoe.

ERIKSON, E. (1950). *Childhood and Society.* New York: Norton.

ERIKSON, E. (1956). The problem of ego identity. *J. of American Psychoanalytic Association,* 4:56-121.

ERIKSON, E. (1962). Reality and actuality. *J. of American Psychoanalytic Association,* 10:451-474.

FREUD, A. (1936). *The Ego and the Mechanisms of Defense.* New York: International Universities Press, 1946.

FREUD, A. (1958). Adolescence. *The Psychoanalytic Study of the Child,* 13:255-278.

INHELDER, B., and PIAGET, J. (1958). *The Growth of Logical Thinking from Childhood to Adolescence.* New York: Basic Books.

JACOBSON, E. (1964). *The Self and the Object World.* New York: International Universities Press.

RIOCH, M. (1970). The work of Wilfred Bion on groups. *Psychiatry,* 33:56-66.

SHAPIRO, E., ZINNER, J., SHAPIRO, R., BERKOWITZ, D. (In press). The influence of family experience on borderline personality development. *Int. Rev. Psychoanalysis.*

SHAPIRO, R. (1963). Adolescence and the psychology of the ego. *Psychiatry.* 26:77-87.

SHAPIRO, R. (1967). The origin of adolescent disturbances in the family: Some considerations in theory and implications for therapy. In *Family Therapy and Disturbed Families.* G. Zuk and I. Boszormenyi-Nagy, eds. Palo Alto: Science and Behavior Books.

SHAPIRO, R. (1968). Action and family interaction in adolescence. In *Modern Psychoanalysis.* J. Marmor, ed. New York: Basic Books.

SHAPIRO, R. (1969). Adolescent ego autonomy and the family. In *Adolescence*: *Psychosocial Perspectives.* G. Caplan and S. Lebovici, eds. New York: Basic Books.

SHAPIRO, R. and ZINNER, J. (In press). Family organization and adolescent development. In *Task and Organization.* E. Miller, ed. London: Tavistock Publications.

TURQUET, P. (1971). Four lectures: *The Bion Hypothesis*: *The Work Group and the Basic Assumption Group.* Given at the National Institute of Mental Health, May 26, May 28, June 2, June 6, 1971.

ZINNER, J., and SHAPIRO, R. (1972). Projective identification as a mode of perception and behavior in families of adolescents. *Int. J. Psychoanalysis,* 53:523-529.

ZINNER, J., and SHAPIRO, R. (1974). The family group as a single psychic entity: Implications for acting out in adolescence. *Int. Rev. Psychoanalysis.* 1:No. 1-2.

ZINNER, J., and SHAPIRO, E. (1974). Splitting in families of borderline adolescents. *Seminars on Psychiatry,* 6, 1, 1974.

7

Office Network Therapy with Adolescents

MAX SUGAR, M.D.

How to best utilize those companions that adolescents bring into the office waiting room with them has always been intriguing. Most frequently an effort is made to extend some amicable greeting to them whether they are relatives or unknown friends, but then it is often unclear what, if anything, to do beyond that. If they are viewed as part of the patient's social network, thereby having some particular potent and specific meaning for the patient and being somehow intertwined with his dynamics, the therapist may then tap this potential field of information for the exposition of his patient's dynamics and for therapy. In this chapter a particular mode of using these companions for specific purposes in the adolescent's therapy will be described.

Speck (1965) coined the phrase "network therapy" to describe his use of the patient's social network. Like others, he had been concerned about the hidden puppeteer behind the scenes, the important key person in the patient's life who never attended the evaluation or family therapy sessions. For adult patients he arranged vertical networks consisting of multi-generations involved with the designated patient in the family's living room. For the adolescent he set up horizontal networks or adolescent peer networks in some large suitable place such as a gym, where family members were not in attendance. The result was a great deal of communication and dynamics about hidden key people in the family.

In family therapy sessions, fear of reprisal may often cause material to be withheld. Also, fear of exposure, shifts in power or status, and other such considerations sometimes lead to abrupt termination of family therapy (Ackerman, 1958).

Langsley and Kaplan (1968) described an approach to crisis with team treatment by which they avoided the hospitalization of the designated patient. They met with that person and his whole family in on-the-spot family therapy in the home or the emergency room for as many sessions as were needed to deal with the crisis on an around-the-clock basis.

There are youngsters who might benefit from group therapy, but their distrust, anxieties about exposure, embarrassment, and ability to control their own impulses in such a setting keep them from it. When a crisis is imminent, it would be unwise to have such a youngster enter a therapy group. If he is already in an adolescent therapy group then certainly he might utilize that setting to deal with the additional conflicts.

I have utilized network therapy with adolescents in an office setting, in private practice, for several specific purposes. One of these is to deal with an imminent crisis which might otherwise eventuate in further disorganization and hospitalization, or a suicidal act. The other specific utilization has been to deal with a youngster who is not having a crisis but whose resistances in therapy do not seem to be manageable with the usual approaches in individual or group therapy. Network therapy in the office may be used alone or in combination with the other therapies. This arrangement, by contrast with Speck's (1965), might be described as a self-selected peer therapy group; it involves no additional or special space, nor additional therapists.

ARRANGEMENTS

The risks of not hospitalizing a youngster who is suicidal, or in need of immediate hospitalization for severe disorganization, must be very carefully assessed. If there seem to be sufficient controls and cooperation available from his environment, as well as a minimum of such from within himself, then network therapy might be a consideration. Then he is asked whether he would like to have a group or therapeutic club of his own. If he is interested, it is explained to him in detail. If he and his family agree, then self-selected peer group therapy is begun. The youngster is told that he may bring whomever he wishes to his own therapy group and that he may have as many friends as often as he wants. It is explained that they may have significant information about him, which if shared in the sessions may be a significant and helpful contribution.

The sessions are arranged as conveniently as possible for the patient and his peers, so as not to conflict with the school or other regularly scheduled activities. The patient may also need to have his other sessions continued or perhaps decreased. No fee is charged to the peers and the patient's fee remains at the usual rate per individual session. The peers may speak of anything they wish during the sessions. They may even ask for help with some of their problems just as the patient does. The therapist has the usual confidentiality concerning his patient and the patient's friends, but no restriction is placed on the patient or his peers about confidentiality or socializing. It is the patient's responsibility to invite people, to explain how the therapy session works and his reason for wanting them there and to inform them of the time and the place of the session.

When the peers attend the session for the first time they are asked to identify themselves and to discuss briefly their relationship with the patient. The basis of procedure is group process, focused mainly on the patient, which allows the patient and peers to interact with one another, with the therapist observing and commenting according to the needs of the situation.

The number of peer group sessions required to deal with the crisis is usually no more than ten and has varied from one to ten. Subsequently, other previous forms of therapy may be pursued, depending on the patient's needs at that time. On some occasions the patient is unable to bring peers and he has an individual session. The decision as to when he discontinues bringing peers is left up to the patient.

CASE ILLUSTRATIONS

Case I

This patient, in his middle adolescent years, was a chronic school truant, a runaway from home and psychiatric hospitals. He had been treated as an inpatient and an outpatient, with individual and group therapy. He had been threatened with restrictions and shock therapy and had been placed in seclusion while in hospitals. He had been discharged from the State Hospital without much change except that he had learned that if he behaved in a certain way, certain punishments would be forthcoming and he learned to avoid them. There were no arrangements made for his schooling, further trade training or therapy. He appeared to be an apathetic schizophrenic with confusion and perplexity, marked suspiciousness, negativism, and occasional dissociation. He spoke in limited monosylables in response to questions and was unmotivated for outpatient group or individual therapy. His parents were interested in some sort of management or therapy for him but they were not very optimistic. They were not interested in any type of therapy for themselves.

Network therapy was offered to him and he eagerly accepted it. His parents accepted it as well, and details were explained. He became quite enthusiastic, verbal and spontaneous. He asked questions about the limitations on his friends, and specifically about confidentiality. He tested and checked several times to see whether I would accept his friends since his parents had told him to stay away from them because they caused trouble for him.

In the early sessions he and his friends were provocative, testing to see what would happen as a result of their comments which previously had caused trouble in school or with other authorities. They brought up some personal matters which were of concern to them and the sources of some conflict. They gave a good deal of data about the patient's past and current associations with them. Among these friends there were two who were especially objectionable to his parents. It was learned that (contrary to the earlier material indicating that he was their puppet) he suggested wild or daring adventures. If one of them did not restrain him verbally or otherwise, he carried out the risky venture. Subsequently, further data was gathered on this theme and it was interpreted to him that he was giving authority to his friends to approve or disapprove of what he did.

Sometimes his friends were quite helpful and kept him out of danger. One of them even prodded him about getting back to school and doing better in it. He seemed to have someone along regularly who represented some aspect of his dynamics, and the area in which he had conflicts and on which he ambivalently wanted to work.

Marked suspiciousness was displayed towards me in the sixth and seventh sessions, and they made assertions about my power and ability to get certain privileges from his parents for him. In the ninth session his friends interpreted to him that he was "so busy screwing other people, that he feels that everyone is going to screw him" and "he does not realize how distrustful he is all the time." They followed this up with detailed illustrations of how he exploited them and how he could not be trusted. After the tenth session he left town as planned for the summer with the idea of staying with a relative and continuing school there. Continued psychiatric therapy was recommended for him but he and his family felt no need for it at that point.

Subsequently it was learned that he had not stayed in school, but had remained out of the hospital though not settled on vocational plans. He had managed to move out of the parental home without any difficulty with authorities and seemed to be marking time before taking the next step. This may have been due to his marked ambivalence, but in any case he was avoiding trouble as well as hospitalization.

Case II

This youngster, who was in his late teens, was severely depressed and psychotic. He was using a variety of drugs such as marijuana, LSD and "speed." On one occasion he had had an acute drug reaction, and with a great deal of panic he admitted himself to a psychiatric hospital overnight. He was seen thereafter on a regular basis but he felt that his problems were due to the drugs. He had attended college irregularly, was at home irregularly and was uncertain where he would be from one night to the next. He had spoken of a number of friends quite often, and on occasion he had one or two of them in the waiting room when he came in for his session. He seemed to be on the verge of further difficulties which seemed indefinable at the time and he did not seem to be utilizing his individual therapy optimally. It was unclear whether he was on drugs during some of the sessions or whether it was denial that was interfering with his progress.

A self-selected peer therapy group was suggested to him and with great suspiciousness and reluctance he feigned agreement. He continued to come in for his individual sessions as before, but without his friends. One session had been regularly and specifically scheduled for his peer group therapy so that he could ask his friends to attend. Each time he came in during the next month he had a rationalization for not having been able to get anyone, such as, "they promised, but did not come."

Then he began bringing in his friends one at a time. Occasionally he came alone for a session and then resumed the network. He had described one friend as being very hostile to his therapy. When this friend came into the session with him he was very hostile and provocative, and demanded an explanation as to why the patient's idea of moving out of his home had not been accepted by me as being well-founded. It was explained to the patient and his friend that the patient had moved out of his home previously on two occasions prematurely and unsuccessfully, and it did not seem to be the proper time for him to move. His friend then attacked further with more demands, as if he were the patient's attorney in a court of law. The patient suddenly became quite anxious as he thought I was going to physically attack and beat his friend and he felt that he wanted to run out of the room. To him it seemed that his friend and I were having an argument over him and I was like his domineering, dictatorial stepfather who would hurt him, while his friend appeared to be the friendly maternal figure. After he took a self-prescribed Librium capsule he immediately felt better and was able to remain in the session.

Once he brought in a friend whom he had casually known, but the friend was not knowledgeable enough about the patient to help him. He seemed very preoccupied with personal matters.

On another occasion, the patient brought in one of his college instructors and his wife. This instructor had told the patient that he did not need treatment—that he just had a problem with his mother—and he proceeded to detail this in highly theoretical, popular, psychiatric jargon which sounded quite confused and provocative.

In another session the patient brought in several friends who seemed quite ingratiating and attempted to be helpful to him.

In the last session he brought in a well-integrated friend whom he had known since seventh grade, and who was now doing well in college. He indicated that the patient "cut people down" and that he was expert in doing this in a humorous fashion. He said additionally that the patient "cuts people down before they can cut him down and lives by the rule of 'Do unto others and hurt them before they can hurt you.'"

After the tenth session of the peer group, which covered about four months, he decided he did not need it anymore and the group was discontinued. He then began to discuss his peers from time to time, and this data was gradually dealt with. He was able to integrate the information and his reaction to the sessions of network therapy so that his friends who had told him not to continue therapy were seen in another light. He was enraged against the friend who had told him that he should stop therapy and move out on his own, as it was now quite clear to him that he could not manage on his own. This person now reminded him of his stepfather, who was inconsistent, violent, unstable and sadistic. (He also looked like his stepfather.) When the data was interpreted, he remembered further details and even brought up corroborative dream material. For instance, he remembered that this person had borrowed his highly prized record collection and had given it away to another person without the patient's permission. This "friend" had now left the city and his whereabouts were unknown, as were the whereabouts of the record collection.

The college instructor was very friendly to him and invited him to his home for drinks before classes. The patient regularly went out of awe and admiration for the instructor. He got drunk every afternoon, did not attend classes and failed the year. When the patient mildly objected to drinking before classes, the instructor told him that he also was drinking. Only later did he realize that the instructor had already taught his classes for the day while the patient had not yet attended his own classes. The instructor had also told him that his problem was his mother, and that he would like to have intercourse with the patient's mother. This material had been suppressed and denied as it was too close to some of his own, unexpressed, oedipal wishes.

The friend who appeared to have been somewhat of a sponge later became quite obviously so in the patient's material and he was able to express himself and deal with the matter more appropriately. The friend who had been more interested in his own situation than in the patient's also came up for scrutiny. This friend, it turned out, had been actively suicidal, and was hospitalized in a state hospital some weeks after having been in the network session with the patient. This was connected with the patient's guilt, wish to undo and magical thinking connected with a suicide in his family.

His resistance seemed largely connected with his ambivalent and confused identifications stimulated by his friends' statements against continuing therapy, which were similar to comments made by his hated stepfather, while his mother firmly stated her support of his therapy.

Case III

This obese, bright, schizoid college freshman had attempted suicide by wrist-slashing (requiring no sutures). She derogated herself, her family, friends and previous therapists. Her three previous suicidal attempts occurred when she felt that there was nothing else she could do, although her goals were vague. Then she became depressed, after which came suicidal ideas and acts.

The one close attachment to a female high school teacher, of which the family disapproved, ended when this teacher moved and the patient's request to go to college in that area was disapproved. Although she was liked by boys and girls, she avoided most socializing; she liked only one boy in college and dated only occasionally, by choice. Her interest in friendships was short and conflicted since she felt worthless.

She had experimented with drugs and had had some weird "bad trips" with LSD and "pot," but this experimentation had not brought her any improvement with relationships or goals.

After several sessions, during which she seemed to overcome some of her early distrust of, and antagonism to continuing in treatment, she made a suicidal attempt with another wrist-slashing. She could not describe the impulses or the need for this behavior any more clearly than she had previously. She was afraid that she would be asked to leave the college and had bound her dormitory-mates in a pact of secrecy to protect herself and them.

After this suicide attempt, one of her three weekly sessions was selected for network therapy sessions. I explained that she could bring in as many of her friends as she wanted, so that they could help us, and she was told that this would be her therapeutic club. She seemed pleased with the idea, but had a number of questions, indicating some fears about it.

For the peer group session, she brought in a dormitory-mate with whom she had been somewhat friendly, but who had not been involved in the secret pact about the suicidal attempt. This girl seemed to be well-integrated, had goals, dated, and was doing very well in her studies. She was very sympathetic and concerned until halfway through the session. Then she voiced concern, annoyance, chagrin and disgust about the patient's suicidal behavior and questioned her reality-testing and her judgment. The patient became agitated at this and tried to defend herself against her friend, who was now confronting and challenging her. They dealt with this and the patient then felt some support from her friend. Bringing this girl along may have represented a wish to emulate her as an ego-ideal, and a desire to organize at a different level than she had previously enjoyed alone or with her less stable friends.

Following this session, she had some grasp of her impulsivity, and decided she did not want to have any further peer group sessions. She continued therapy and classes until the end of the semester. Although still uncertain about her goals, she did not want to stay at home, and elected to travel until she settled on her own goal, at which time she planned to return and resume therapy.

On follow-up a year later she was not in school but had been traveling and visiting friends. She felt she was managing well but had not decided on any long-term goals. She had lost weight, was slim and well-groomed which made her hard to recognize at first, as this was a marked contrast to her last appearance.

DISCUSSION

Early in adolescence there is a natural tendency for gangs of the same sex to form. In middle adolescence they are transformed to heterosexual groups, but the gangs themselves go through many changes, with frequent shifts in their composition and numbers as their values, interests, ego ideals and narcissistic involvements change along with the adolescent's own changes in various psychic structures and function. The spontaneous group seems to be one of the functional foundations for the self-selected peer group (Richmond and Schechter, 1964).

Among those youngsters who have accepted network therapy there seems to be a fierce loyalty to some of their peers in spite of rather loose associations or the appearance of apathy. This seems to be an indicator that network therapy would be potentially useful and successful since it is related to their level of object relations. For network therapy to be successful with these youngsters it seems that the level of object relations should at least be at the ambivalent level, although it may be fluctuating between the anaclitic and ambivalent levels. This is reflected in the ties to their peers, although in some cases they are dependent on their friends, rather than sharing or cooperating with them. The patients also reflect this in their ties to their parents, which are based on an anaclitic level of object relations, shifting to the symbiotic or ambivalent level. None of them had managed to separate and individuate suitably, although there had been precocious pseudoindependence in some of their behavior. Beneath all this there was an intense symbiotic tie to a parent. This level of object relations is also reflected in the youngster having strong conforming needs for his own subculture.

The adolescent has phase-specific tasks related to sexual and aggressive drive accommodations, psychic structural changes and physical adaptations in an attempt to achieve ordinary adolescent development. Where there are additional strains to the revival of the oedipal and pre-oedipal conflicts in an emotionally ill youngster at a symbiotic or ambivalent level of object relations, the usual therapeutic approaches may be insufficient to manage his difficulties and needs. Complications may occur, such as acting out a psychosis or a neurosis for a parent, excessive guilt feelings, suicidal ideation and behavior, excessive separation anxiety with withdrawal from the environment and clinging to the parents, explosive tantrum-like behavior with violent actions, or other such unsuitable adaptive or defensive efforts. Some of these adolescents may then feel hopeless and attempt suicide or give the therapist the feeling that suicide may seem imminent, or they may become disorganized, behaving in such a way that hospitalization seems to be needed immediately.

When the environment can be minimally cooperative, either of these alternatives may be avoided by the use of the self-selected peer group.

The active cooperation of the parents or guardians, along with their continued support and understanding, as well as contact, is therefore crucial to manage the crisis. The therapy may pose a threat to the parent and the symbiotic child. Therefore every effort should be made not to threaten this tie and to seek the parent's cooperation. Subsequently separation and individuation gradually occur and replace the symbiotic tie to the parent with more suitable developments when therapy is successful.

Adolescents are usually very hostile and unyielding to someone who does not seem to have the behavior or appearance that is acceptable to them and who has not conformed to their expectations. When the patient is allowed to choose his own supporting cast for his therapy group, its members indeed support him, as they are friends or acquaintances whose defenses are acceptable to him. They do not pose a threat to him at that point or to the symbiosis with a parent, although the parents may experience the friends as a threat.

The self-selected therapy group of peers uses the ordinary social situation to enhance the wishes and needs of the patient and his family to separate from each other. This is in reaction to the binds that they impose on each other and is the natural developmental need. When therapy is successful, this develops slowly. Previously the efforts to be rid of one another have led to hospitalization, possibly to suicide attempts or other disturbing behavior.

The self-selected peer group promotes a gradual and controlled therapeutic innoculation or immunization, as well as a therapeutic togetherness from which a simultaneous separation is initiated. The togetherness is built on the basis of a diluted symbiosis with the therapist and peers, which allows the patient to present, expose, discuss, investigate and deal with conflicts more suitably. There is a diluted transference to the therapist and a strong bond with the peers. This inaugurates some separation from the family. Ultimately the ties with the therapist and family decrease while the bonds with peers may remain for as long as the patient needs the particular peers. This tie to peers leads to a peer symbiosis which helps increase and promote barriers to the family symbiosis, thus assisting in the separation-individuation process.

In offering the patient network therapy, the therapist reflects some possibilities for the adolescent's increased autonomy and self-esteem as well as some responsibility for himself. The appeal to his healthy islands of ego functioning raises his self-esteem as the patient is asked to be in charge of himself and his friends. Simultaneously, the therapist is indicating approval of his ties to his peers. The patient is also asked to make some choices in a particular, specific, limited situation. Eventually he becomes more responsible as this provides a stimulus for some controls by himself and his autonomy. This indicates some respect for the patient as an individual, as he is asked to use his own judgment and make some decisions on his own. The youngster may be introjecting the therapist, and the omnipotence ascribed by him to the therapist to do this initially.

The frequency with which certain friends are brought in may provide significant clues to the therapist as to some of the dynamics and level of therapy that the patient is able to work with during that particular session. The choice of provocative, psychopathic, or psychotic peers may indicate resistance. The therapist's own awareness of this test of trust, or the effort to provoke may be crucial in managing the resistance.

The material that is brought in of this nature is available for all parties to examine immediately or subsequently in the network or later in individual therapy if this is needed. For example, with the second case, one friend was a thief and persuaded the patient to assist him in grand larceny. He promoted paranoid ideas in the patient who feared that he would be exposed or reported to the police, even though the events had transpired years earlier when he was quite young. As he was able to discuss this exploitative friend many months later, further material came up related to the network session. It was amazing how the patient was now able to bring into focus this material that his observing ego had carefully stored away and integrate it with the current evaluation of his friends and himself.

It should be noted that the patient may unconsciously be using an antisocial, exploitative, or psychotic friend to focus on his own similar traits. The frequency with which certain peers attend gives a further clue to the direction of the therapy, since their productions, memories and interpretations to the patient will have a particular theme and relevance. The presence of a psychotic peer in one instance seemed related to the patient's wish to see some of his own abnormal behavior through the reflection of his friend, as well as to display some of his healthy islands of ego function.

In network therapy the issue of the youngster associating with the wrong kind of friends does not come up except as material showing how bad the parents are, which is a complaint by the patient and his friends to the therapist. The therapist's acceptance of all the patient's peers is an important test for the therapist. It is also a crucial reflection of what the youngster is struggling with developmentally, and may be a source of conflict within himself and with his family.

It is particularly noteworthy that some of the peers begin to function like parents at some point. Initially they may be quite supportive, sympathetic and accepting of all that the patient says. Regardless of whether they themselves are well-integrated, they frequently bring up and confront the patient with his unrealistic attitudes or destructive behavior. Thus they often express their concern for him and his maladaptive behavior. On first hearing such comments the patient experiences it as an onslaught and then turns to the therapist for support. Such confrontations or interpretations by peers are often quite effective since hearing it from a peer makes it seem much more real and honest and cannot be dismissed as a parental complaint. The patient seems to be caught off-guard with his defensive barrier lowered since the peer is present at his request and as a favor to him. Thus, no verbal assault is expected. Frequently he does not ask this peer back again, but if he does it is several weeks later. Such an event seems to herald a crisis of improved integration and it is usually managed between the patient and the peers without the therapist intervening. Usually in one or two sessions after such a crisis the patient indicates that he has no further need of the network for therapy.

SUMMARY

Office network therapy, or the self-selected peer therapy group, has been used successfully as an adjunct to deal with a critical situation to avoid a suicide attempt or hospitalization, as well as to deal with some major resistances in one to ten sessions. For some youngsters in such crises, neither individual, family nor group therapy seems to be feasible, although these modalities have been combined with network therapy with other patients.

The peers chosen are usually better integrated than the patient although some of them may be as disturbed emotionally as the patient. There is a potential for a diluted tie with the peers which may be apparent from an intense positive bond with them. The peers selected may be particular indicators diagnostically and therapeutically of the patient's readiness to focus on certain conflicted areas. Inviting peers who are questionable from the parents' standpoint may be a very meaningful test of trust of the therapist, as well as being related to efforts at autonomy and improved self-esteem on the patient's part. This becomes especially significant in connection with the patient's symbiotic ties with the parents and the needs for separation and individuation which have not been completed.

Network therapy seems to be most easily accepted by adolescents who have a strong need to conform with their own subculture. This seems to reflect their level of object relations as they have a need for conformity and clinging, since their ties with their peers are at an anaclitic, or symbiotic, or ambivalent level. If the parents are cooperative and supportive the venture has a much greater chance of being successful.

REFERENCES

ACKERMAN, N. W. (1958). *The Psychodynamics of Family Life.* New York: Basic Books.

LANGSLEY, D. G., and KAPLAN, D. M. (1968). *The Treatment of Families in Crisis.* New York: Grune and Stratton.

RICHMOND, A. H., and SCHECTER, S. (1964). A spontaneous request for treatment by a group of adolescents. *Int. J. Group Psychother.,* 14:97-106.

SPECK, R. V. (1965). Psychotherapy of the social network of a schizophrenic family. *Family Process,* 5:204-214.

8

Defusing a High School Critical Mass

Max Sugar, M.D.

The widely publicized social and educational turbulence in American colleges and high schools in the 1960's has been described as a mirror reflecting the foreign and domestic behavior of our government (Schrag, 1971). Anthony (1970) made a parallel statement that every generation gets the kind of adolescents it deserves.

The increase in revolutionary tendencies in colleges, as well as the militancy in senior and even junior high schools, may reflect any one, or a combination, of the following: serious intrapsychic conflict in the adolescents involved; a sociologic upheaval; a reaction against a suppressive and destructive phenomenon at the upper echelon of bureaucracy and government; or a reaction against a phenomenon in these echelons that is in transition, disjointed, and anxiety-ridden, the anxiety filtering down from adults to adolescents.

Various modes of dealing with these reactions have been described. Rueveni (1971) used a sensitivity training method with 15 students. Anshin (1970), who met with faculty, parents, and students separately to assess their views, established an open-ended therapeutic group for the students. Schnell and associates (1970) organized four committees from among parents, students and faculty of a high school, which led to a common effort at communicating and solving problems.

The present report concerns the successful management of a critical situation in a high school which was on the verge of a violent eruption in 1970-71, according to school authorities. Among factors considered are the background of this school, how racial polarization had created an explosive situation, major transitions in the school administration, exploitation of the school by outsiders for profit, and disequilibrium among adults in the school. The use of group process in a forum to deal with the situation will be described, as well as the transitional developments and their effects on the adolescents. Specific comments about individual dynamics cannot be made, since there was no effort at history-taking, individual assessment, or therapy.

THE HIGH SCHOOL

The population of the high school was long established as white male and predominantly middle class until it became coeducational in 1951 and then biracial in the mid-sixties. Reaction to the racial integration was prejudiced fear, mainly that the intrusion of blacks, with their socio-economic and educational disadvantages, would damage the school's social, academic and athletic lustre.

In 1968-69, the school had had many types of difficulties: polarization between the races; authority problems; monetary extortion of students by other students; frequent threats to, and assaults on teachers and students by students and outsiders. Drugs were easily obtained inside and outside the school, and many students were "stoned" during classes. During a three-day student strike, based on demands made by some militant black students with outside help, many students paraded around the school with placards and did not attend classes; others were absent because they feared for their safety. After the strike, classes resumed, and a community action committee began to study the situation and make recommendations. What they arrived at seemed to be a bland *non culpa* decision about all the authorities involved and a mild chastisement of the students. Later, there was shooting by police at outsiders who invaded the school.

Academic 1969-70 saw similar events except for the absence of a strike. An increased tempo of fear, anxiety, and trauma led the faculty to consider building a protective fence around the school with locked gates. The faculty compromised with the parents by having unarmed guards at all exits during school hours during the latter half of the year. The remoteness, rigidity, and inaccessibility of the principal made his rumored retirement of several years seem like the solution to the school's problems. In the summer of 1970, he retired without any prior announcement to the faculty or students.

The officers of the Parent-Teacher Association were extremely concerned that violence would erupt when the new principal took over. There were forebodings that he would act restrictively and that the resultant pressures would increase student difficulties. Additionally, the faculty was uncertain how he would function in his new role as their superior rather than their peer. The problems in the school seemed to be related to the usual adolescent range of difficulties, plus apprehension about the new principal, racial polarization, student-teacher polarization, and lack of a stimulating curriculum, especially for students who were not college-bound. Since the school had no psychiatric consultation, the officers of the PTA sought help from private volunteer psychiatrists. After several preparatory meetings, the forum started.

THE FORUM

A forum based on a group approach was offered to all students, parents, faculty, and teachers connected with the high school. This was not designed as a therapy or action group but rather was aimed at increasing communication and sharing, and understanding by discussion. No effort was to be made to uncover any of the students' emotional problems. Because of the polarization, there was increasing isolation and tension, and it was felt that improved communication might at least give an opportunity to air some of the problems, differences and grievances, and perhaps reduce some of the tensions.

The principal was notified of these plans and his cooperation was sought. In the preliminary meeting with the school principal and vice principal before the first forum, the issues were presented to them, as well as to invited group leaders, in as diplomatic, non-competitive, helpful, and kindly a fashion as possible. The principal was very tense about the matter, although he seemed to grasp the essence of the issue and the potential positives involved. He viewed the forum as a threat to his authority and leadership. Before leaving, he delivered a kind of pep talk to the group leaders and officers of the PTA, stressing the importance of virtue.

The forum was publicized through announcements on the public address system of the school several days before and again on the day of each meeting, by distribution of mimeographed invitations provided by the PTA to each student to take home to parents, by announcements in the PTA Newsletter, and by placards posted in conspicuous places around the school.

Six group leaders, all of them mental health professionals experienced in group process and therapy, acted as assistant leaders for the forum. The author acted as the forum leader. All participants gathered in a large circle in the cafeteria in the basement of the high school. After a 15-

minute introductory large group session, small groups met in the classrooms, with chairs arranged in a circle. They confronted one another and conversed for an hour, under the guidance and leadership of the one or two professionals in the group. They then reassembled as a full group. After a summary was presented by a student or other spokesman chosen by each group, there was a discussion with questions and answers for another 15 to 30 minutes. Then the group leaders met briefly to discuss the developments from a professional viewpoint. This meeting was attended by the principal and assistant principal.

An effort at neutralization was introduced whereby, although no confidentiality was offered, no retribution would be forthcoming for statements made in these sessions. The participants were not required to remain in the same group at every meeting. This was done in order to reduce the transference involvements with the leaders and keep the forum from becoming a therapy group. The forum was to be communicative, ventilative, and abreactive, but not investigative and not designed to deal with the intrapsychic conflicts or dynamics of the participants.

The forum was held in the evenings at the school, instead of an unfamiliar place, in order to make students, faculty, and parents feel more at ease. It was decided to limit attendance to those students, parents, and faculty directly involved with the high school since invasion by outsiders for personal profit was part of the problem.

THE FORUM MEETINGS

Some highlights of the sessions are presented here.

Session 1

About 120 parents, students, teachers and faculty attended the first session. The forum leader spent 15 minutes explaining the arrangements of, and hopes for the forum. The group was reassured that this was not going to be therapy nor was it a probing into their heads; their conversations were to be entirely voluntary; they were not being asked to confess and they need not fear later punishment, retaliation or discipline by the school or parents for any of their statements; here they could feel free to express their complaints, questions, and problems, and have a meaningful exchange of ideas. The full group then divided into six smaller groups of about 20 each and chose a leader. (The basis for this choice was never established.)

The students aired many valid grievances. They first asked for details about how the forum would work, what the goals were, and what action would be instituted by the group leaders. They raised questions about school rules, some of which had been instituted recently by the new principal to regain control of the school and included restrictions about lunch times and gathering places on the street before and after school. They asked about courses that had been discontinued shortly after school began. There were many complaints directed at specific teachers.

With the many grievances directed at the principal, he became very anxious and often defended himself with authoritative, emotional statements. At other times, however, he was able to explain to the students why certain rules were being changed and others were being instituted, and why some courses were no longer being offered. These explanations seemed to reassure the students. They learned that decisions were not made simply on a whim of the authorities, but on the basis of some real thought and effort.

The students and their own parents had many bellicose exchanges, which represented an extension of the arguments at home. At times students sided with the embattled parents, at others with the students. Some of the complaints were resolved when some new slant or view was offered to help clarify the situation and place it in a more objective light. The summaries presented at the end of the meeting led to a broadening of the complaints, explanations, and understanding of them as well as their universalistic nature. The suggestion was made to bring to the next forum peers who were completely satisfied with the school.

The principal entered the post-forum meeting with the leaders and stayed in spite of not having been invited or being made to feel especially welcome at first. Nevertheless, the discussion continued, and although technical terms were used sparingly, certain explanations were made to the principal so that he would know what was being discussed. His anxiety at this point was high because he was a prime target, and because he was uncomfortable about being with professionals and not understanding everything they "were doing to his school."

Session 2

Of the 100 people in attendance at the second session, about half were students. Considerable hostility was expressed against all the authorities in the school—the principal, school nurse, vice principal, counselors, as well as Student Council members. Other complaints included discontinuation of the school paper, preferential treatment for seniors, and reduction in physical education classes from five to three times weekly. The students were also disturbed about the school's reputation, now being known as a "cop-out school where students who couldn't make it anywhere else can pass."

There were problems in communication; some were not listening to or did not hear others, and there were interruptions and misunderstandings. When this was pointed out there were fewer interruptions and a greater effort to understand others rather than simply griping and yelling.

The principal was again the target for strong hostile feelings, partly of a transference nature and partly related to reality issues about his administration. The students attacked his controlling things so tightly that they felt "jailed." At the end of the second session, he seemed more upset than after the first. He stated that he might not attend further sessions because the students seemed to be focusing on him alone and not discussing other issues that he considered needed airing. He was offered some reassurance and support, with an explanation of the transference phenomenon. The importance of his presence to the success of the forums was stressed insofar as the students were learning to communicate with him.

In the first two sessions there seemed to be a good deal of orality, oral sadism, and hostility, with many side and cross conversations with interruptions. These were discussed to point up the need to listen to the other person, and to respect the ideas of others even if they disagreed. In the second session the biting comments were mixed with some efforts at control on the part of the students; they expressed their anality through their wish to destroy everything in operation and introduce new rules with them in control. The usual adolescent rebellion and reaction-formation were obvious in the desire to break all the rules and attack all hypocrisy and all authority and to replace it with something new which they had devised themselves.

At an "open house" at the school between the second and third sessions there was considerable optimism, the result in part of the cheerful new colors used to paint the school during the summer. The parents stayed and talked together after the meeting until 10:30 p.m., instead of leaving immediately as they had previously. The teachers also stayed for the first time. The additional enthusiasm seemed attributable to the fact that a large number of parents met and communicated for the first time in the forum.

The third meeting was held one week after the second.

Session 3

The forum leader opened the discussion with a reference to the growing optimism in the school and some indications of positively developing communication. The smaller groups discussed problems in communication, the small numbers of students attending, and better publicity for the forum in order to increase attendance.

In this session there was a continuance of the gripes and demands that had been voiced in the two previous sessions, with desires for restitution, complaints from the seniors about what they had not obtained in their first two years in high school, about the school's indifference to the students' requests, and about the limitations on their lunch and pleasure time.

Four groups of about 15 per group brought the attendance to 60. Three of the leaders were absent. There was some discussion about the absence of the student leaders, members of the Student Council. More blacks were present in the third session, and more students than adults for the first time.

The students expressed a good deal of ambivalence about their education and their goals, and blamed the teachers for not stimulating them, although they admitted not having any sustained goals, "freaking out" or playing hookey and needing vocational training. They were not able to relate this to their ambivalence and displacement to teachers.

In the large group discussion there was further development of the issues in the small groups. The rage, hate, and projection had decreased and a positive feeling about the school and the forum had begun to appear. A white male student brought up the question of the spontaneous black-white segregation, which was evident not only in the school but in the forum as well. The absence of some parents was noted and the author commented that perhaps communication was better between parents and students in families where parents attended the forum.

At this forum, in the middle of October, there was less tension and more enthusiasm and optimism among the students, and the polarities seemed to have lessened somewhat.

Session 4

The fourth session was in early November. There were about 40 participants, most of whom were students. The principal and assistant principal were present, as were some parents, but no teachers. Two group leaders were absent. The group leaders doubled up and co-led three groups, in which they discussed the police picking up students in the park. The blacks were arguing among themselves about the cops as "pigs" and talked about provoking authority rather than avoiding fights. The blacks monopolized the group while the white students primarily watched. Having observed a strange stream of conversation by several blacks, the forum leader suggested a change in seating to intervene in the pairing and make the discussion broader for all present. Discussion then centered on the Student Council representatives who were the good students in the school but who were not present; they looked down on the others, and those present returned the feeling. The students spoke of wanting controls from the principal, but also of not wanting such controls. The author confronted them with several observations: that three conversations were going on at the same time with no speaker listening or respecting the others' comments; that the students did not listen to adults or to each other; that they seemed to disrespect each other; and that they didn't listen to the problems they had in common. He stressed their common problems and those they had in communication.

In this session the blacks were difficult to understand, as their enunciation was unclear and listening to them became fatiguing. At first it seemed related to their deprived background and difficulty in speaking in a large group. Their speech content semed to be provocative and hostile, but as they clarified themselves in better English, it became apparent they were speaking in the dialect that they use only among themselves. This suggested a further decrease in distrust and an increase in communication among the blacks, who were more openly assertive and hostile.

The blacks feared that the homecoming dance would not be successful because it was not being supported by the whites. At the dance the previous year one black male had stabbed another. There seemed to be some increased openness, trust, spontaneity, and sharing, with less guardedness and suspicions among those present.

Session 5

The fifth session, which was held two weeks after the fourth, was attended by only 32 people. The small attendance seemed related to the trimester examinations held that week, another parents' meeting at the same time, and the PTA meeting the next night.

One of the students suggested at the full meeting that one topic be discussed each night. The author replied that the forum was an open one available for the discussion of any subject and his idea opposed the very foundation of the forum. He was also told that he could discuss this in his small group if he wished.

He and a friend chose to be in the author's group for the third consecutive time, and suggested that the topic for the night be "pigs-police." Some students shifted the discussion to the difficulty in getting first aid from the school nurse. The folk festival was brought up as a way for people to get to know one another, but this event had until now been fostered and promoted by black students, with little positive response from whites.

When the group leader asked one of the young ladies who had been silent about her thoughts, she responded that she was not connected with the school, but was only the older sister of one of the students present. She was asked to leave the forum because it was open only to students, parents, teachers, and faculty. Her brother angrily challenged the leader about the rules and threatened to retaliate later. The leader repeated the initial agreement about the forum, but this student continued to needle, quiz, and provoke the leader.

Later in the large group, the forum discussed the homecoming dance, the folk festival, and the rules about outsiders not being present. One of the group leaders, who supported the students' wish to invite outsiders, seemed to be sabotaging the effects of the total forum. Fourteen persons admitted having brought in outsiders at one time or another through misunderstanding, defiance, or ignorance. The more vocal, militant members of the forum wanted to have a committee to decide about a rule change, but the forum leader declined and referred the question to the small groups for discussion.

One of the students then vocalized his wish that the students be included in the planning and be represented on the leaders' committee. Again the leader referred the question to small group discussion.

To avoid a conflict with other school events, the principal was to notify the PTA President about free dates. The forum leader's suggestion that the next meeting be held four weeks hence was accepted. There was obvious resistance side by side with positive effects of the forum and a negative transference shift to the forum leader from the principal.

Some students had selected the same group leader for three or four consecutive sessions, and both positive and negative transferences, therefore, were apparently being furthered, as well as the tendency to therapy, by the close frequency of meetings and the regular attendance of the forum leader. The other leaders had variable attendance. For this reason, the forum leader decided not to attend the next meeting and requested that one of the other group leaders chair it. The principal, several weeks later, notified the President of the PTA of the date of the next meeting, and she, in turn, notified the forum leaders and the students.

In the post-forum session the leader mentioned to the other group leaders that the defiance and the provocation about issues and rules by several of the students were related to transference displaced from the principal and parents to the forum leader. Two of the group leaders agreed with the chairman of the forum, but the other two did not and objected to a discussion or analysis of the process. They just wanted the students to have a voice in the planning of the forum, which they thought should be open to all outsiders. The principal pointed out, however, that the forum was sponsored by the school and was for the school, not for outsiders. The two dissenting group leaders were in a major transitional turmoil because of impending job changes to other cities, as was learned three months later when they did not attend further meetings. After the meeting the principal indicated his awareness of the transference phenomenon when he jokingly suggested that he might "take the heat off" the forum leader by angering the students somehow.

Session 6

The sixth session was held in January, 1971, allowing a cooling-off period of two months for dilution of some feelings. The 24 participants consisted of eleven students, four teachers, three parents, five group leaders, and the principal. It was decided to meet in one large group for that evening. Some parents questioned the wisdom of holding classes at the beginning and end of the school year when books are unavailable for several weeks. The principal explained that a specific number of school attendance days were required of each student, regardless of whether books were available or not. The discussion led to questions of what education is about, what the problems in learning are, whether students need a teacher with a program to be learning, and about alternative learning experiences.

The students contended that they were not given enough opportunity to be heard, but the teachers argued that some teachers are better qualified to handle discussion groups than others and that students need to learn how to listen and respect one another. This had been an issue throughout the forum when the students interrupted one another, their parents, and teachers, or shouted in an effort to command respect. Some of the discussion then centered on the need to avoid manipulating. The growth in the group was indicated by the students' desire to clean up the school patio and to plant some trees under which they could sit and hold open discussions. The following Saturday some 50 students voluntarily cleaned up the school patio.

The students were now extending their interests beyond the school curriculum and rules to the outside world and doing something about it themselves. They had become involved in discussions about sex and drugs. Now they were interested in cleaning up the environment, as indicated by their behavior in cleaning up the school patio. They were now actively defusing their school and environment.

Session 7

This session, one month later, was attended by three black students, four white students, three group leaders, and two parents. The principal was attending another school function, but sent a message that there were no special problems except for some minor trouble with non-student outsiders still coming into the school.

Two black students, new to the forum, raised the question of their acceptability in the group since they were only sophomores and most of the other students were seniors. There was a discussion about the status of seniors connected with imminent changes in the school hierarchical system. This was the first expression of the seniors' separation anxiety over leaving school to go to work or to college. They discussed the adjustment necessary in progressing from junior high school to senior high school and from senior high to college.

There was considerable discussion about the lack of communication, with a focus on the hypocrisy of the principal who "talks nice only when scared and talks only to one student at a time." They raised questions about: why the school quadrangle was not used after it had been cleaned; why chains were kept on the doors to the outside of the building; what the function of the nurse in the school was, since she was so difficult to get to see; how to get out of school when one is sick since the nurse will not allow a sick student to go home or go to see his own doctor if she cannot reach the parents by telephone; why the public address system was not working; why the teachers were allowed to be absent so much; why rules are not imposed on teachers; why the teachers and students were apathetic. The grievances expressed by the group were more realistic, but their rebellious feelings and problems with authority were obvious. This may have been explained by the long gap between sessions which were now a month apart.

Because of the small number, this session was managed as one group. The students—blacks and whites—seemed to be somewhat closer to one another, discussed issues more freely, and showed greater unity than previously. Problems of communication continued to be pointed out; questions were raised about how information should be disseminated to the students.

After the forum session was over that night, the forum leader met the principal on his way out, and the principal seemed in high spirits. He had received, at the other function, a positive response from the students. He considered the evening a success and apologized for his absence from the forum.

Session 8

The eighth session, held a month later, was attended by seven students, two parents, the principal, a faculty member responsible for student affairs, and one group leader. The presence of an outsider, the older brother of a student, did not hold much interest for the participants. The low attendance at the forum was owing to the competition from an important boxing match held that night. The PTA President reported that the students were glad that the forum was being held even though most did not attend. Questions about curriculum changes were raised but mostly desultory issues were brought up. The student affairs faculty member supported the militant, provocative comments made by one of the students.

One bright student raised the question about the unstimulating classroom teaching. The principal responded with a very long discussion, finally agreeing that the complaint was justified, but pointing out the students' needs for some self-responsibility. The student, who had been most articulate, demanding, and militant in previous meetings, requested a special talk on social injustices in the high school and complained that the forum never resulted in positive action. The PTA President pointed out that positive action had been taken as a result of the forum. The feeling was that the tone of the forum had changed from anger and defiance to dissent over apathy and boredom among the students.

The next forum was scheduled to be held a month later. The day before this meeting occurred, the special faculty member in charge of student affairs, the ombudsman, took over the function of the forum without consultation with the forum leader or the PTA President. The forum was then discontinued. The ombudsman had started having meetings with the students in the gym during school hours because of the small number of students attending the forum recently. The school was now having a forum on its own. The forum leader, other group leaders, and the PTA President gave a great deal of encouragement, support, and explanation to the principal throughout the year.

RESULTS

The decrease in attendance from an initial average of 100 participants to 15 in the later forums indicated that there was a decreased need for, and interest in the forum. The school had been defused as though it had been an active bomb about to blow up; the forum had thus been successful in managing the crisis. There were only ten fights during the school year among the biracial, coeducational student body of 1800. This was a relatively small number, considering the interracial and interpersonal problems. Some of the students, who in the previous year had looked for fights, were now hardworking and doing very well in their classes. The school was now able to manage without the forum since there was no longer any crisis.

A further positive result of the forum was that the Student Council in January, 1971, during Student Council Week, had divided the students into groups of 20 during the daily gym period and held their own forum with a Student Council member as a monitor. This was done without teachers, faculty, or parents. The discussions in the small groups were presented in summary form to the large group at the end. Out of these sessions, led by the Student Council members, emerged plans for improving the school, dealing with the principal's rules, and solving other school problems. It led to the discussion of pleasant, shared school activities, such as originating and planning the school carnival at the end of the school year. Thus, another one of the original goals of the forum had also been attained: some of the Student Council members, who had not been greatly interested or represented in the forum meetings but had attended infrequently, had taken over another part of the forum through identification and imitation.

Emulating the forum leaders' approach to understanding, the Student Council arranged a "drug room" in the school in the spring to handle students' drug problems, by giving information about getting medical help. It therefore seemed that they had had a positive experience from the forum and had been able to identify for the first time with a concerned adult. They learned to listen, to respect the others' feelings and thoughts, to communicate, and to convert their needs into something positive and constructive.

There had been some unification among the students, as well as students and faculty, with fewer barriers between them. The school principal was commended highly by the School Board for his successful school year and given a promotion. The assistant principal, a black who had attended the forum meetings, became the acting principal. He was supported by the parents for the position "because he had been with us through it all."

DISCUSSION

The early sessions of the forum were on a demand basis; the frequency was set by a vote of the group. At first they were mostly gripe sessions with a great deal of demanding, sarcasm, and rage, which partly masked the intense dependency needs and conflict. Complaints were directed particularly at the school principal, the curricula, play time, lunch time, teachers, and counselors. Hence, it was a phase of dependency and symbiotic conflicts.

In the second, or middle phase, the sessions were directed more towards the level of controls, and ambivalence was the highlight. In the next few meetings, discussions became less concerned with complaints about the school personnel and curriculum and were directed more to external matters, such as festivals, sex, drugs, police, getting "busted," and fears about the school carnival and dance. The fact that the language of the black dialect was heard indicated some assertiveness on the part of the blacks and reflected elements of defiance and trust, letting the white man know this, shutting him out, but clarifying when asked.

There was a challenging of authority about the rules and one demonstration in the large group about outsiders not being welcome. There were threats and dares made to the leader of the forum about students being excluded from leadership functions. Attendance dropped from the early phase, when it was 100 to 30-60 in the middle phase. There was resistance side by side with observable positive effects, along with a negative transference shift from the principal to the forum leader.

In the later phase attendance dropped to an average of 15 per meeting. Whereas the meetings were less intense, there was more open communication, some unity among students, concern about the students' apathy and boredom, as well as somewhat more autonomous functioning among the students. The senior students had some rising tension about their separation from school with their graduation at the end of April. In this phase, besides identifying with, they also learned from interested adults who listened and tried to help them deal with the issues of importance through abreaction, ventilation, discussion, universalization, explanation, clarification, and redirection, rather than impulsive or destructive action or withdrawal. There was some slightly decreased ambivalence about the adult world with some increased self-responsibility and further separation from the infantile objects. This was also indicated by the decreased parental and teacher attendance. There was great accommodation to feelings of revenge, anger, and loss of the former principal, acceptance of the new one, as well as each of the different races. The teachers may have had some decreased anxiety about their role vis-à-vis the new principal.

POWER ATTRIBUTION

Lippitt, Polansky, Redl, and Rosen (1958) noted that a "group member is more likely to imitate the behavior of those members to whom he attributes high power in the group . . . (and) is more likely to accept the induction attempts of members with high attributed power."

Although it was explained that the forum was not an action group, and that the forum leaders did not have any power, there was obviously some imputation thereof. The principal, assistant principal, some counselors, and teachers attended the forum, where they became visible to the students and parents for hostile, verbal barrages and confrontations. Decisions in the forum, such as frequency of meetings, were not made by the school administration but by the group under the forum leaders' guidance. The induction of fair play, majority rule, and democratic process was heeded by all present. Infractions of the basic arrangements were brought up by the forum leader for discussion. When it was learned that the principal and two of the group leaders brought in outsiders (their young children, for the sake of convenience), their position of power may have seemed lessened and more power attributed to the forum leader.

It seems likely that the power attributed to the mental health professionals may have been a factor in the acceptance by the participants of the implied help with, and hope for resolution of the difficulties within the school. Additionally, this may have contributed to the students' listening to the nondirective efforts to improve communication and ultimately to imitate and identify with the group leaders and have their own sessions modeled after the forum.

The group leaders aimed at understanding the adolescent with a non-omnipotent modesty. Many times the response to students' questions was "I don't know, but what are your ideas?" One reason the students attended at first was to validate their belief that no adult cared for or believed them. They challenged the group leaders to be honest. When the group leaders were found to be credible, the students gained a modicum of confidence in adults, which was then transferred to the school authorities. Doubtless, this was aided by the principal and other adults giving straight answers.

PREJUDICE AND SOCIAL CHANGE

Prejudice and social changes seem to have been of central significance in this high school. Prejudice is often explained as a projection of one's own undesirable traits. Bettelheim and Janowitz (1964) stated that downward social mobility operates to increase ethnic prejudice and intolerance and that:

> prejudice in the lower status groups is usually greater than in the middle status groups. . . . Ethnic hostility and prejudice are part of a particularistic way of life which protects the continued existence of social units by binding them even more closely together, and by inuring them against universalistic tendencies. . . . Prejudice facilitates the discharge of hostility, and if hostility is discharged, anxiety is reduced.
>
> If prejudice can bolster a weak sense of identity, the loss of this psychological supportive mechanism may threaten a weak identity. Efforts at racial integration threaten not only the social status and economic security of a prejudiced group, but actually the inner sense of identity of its members. Steps toward integration mean criticism of their prejudices—a criticism that increases certain guilt feelings they may be unable to admit even to themselves. As a result, they may feel psychologically trapped, because now both criticism and guilt threaten their sense of identity. . . . Ethnic prejudice is always a group phenomenon.

The forum gave the participants an opportunity to express their hostility verbally to the other race and generation, thus reducing some of their anxiety. The prejudice here was from multiple sources: youth to parents and school authorities; parents to offspring; principal to students, parents and teachers; teachers to principal, students and parents; black to white; male to female. Universalizing in the group and making one participant's difficulty a focus of concern for all, even if only temporarily, introduced commonality which had a unifying effect—feeling oneself part of the larger group of humans with problems. This may have indirectly aided in the reduction of prejudices, although they did not disappear, as indicated by the complaints about black-white prejudice and avoidance of the homecoming dance.

TRANSITIONAL FACTORS

If there is a concatenation of traumatic events which overwhelm the available defenses, maladaptive behavior, symptomatic of this, occurs. This applies especially to children and adolescents. In this school, at the time the forum began, the school racial composition was in transition and a new principal entered the scene.

During a transition period, there may be a tendency toward crises. Whether situational or accidental, when a stress is superimposed on a normal developmental crisis, the combined impact of these simultaneous events may lead to a crisis of major proportions.

The change in the racial and sexual composition of the student body put the school in some quandary about its tradition as an all-boy, white, middle-class school, with a history of great successes athletically and high standards of academic excellence. The incoming black students with deprived educational and economic backgrounds posed a threat of lowering of the school standards. The racial change was more threatening to the middle-class parents and students than the coeducational change which had been introduced some dozen years before.

Added to this was a transition involving imminent retirement of the principal of many years. Although he stayed on, the following year the rumors of this retirement increased. More militancy, extortions, drug peddling, absenteeism, threats, and assaults on teachers and students, as well as invasion by outsiders, occurred. Guards were hired, and there was talk of building a fence to keep outsiders out, to manage fear of a further explosion.

The question of the principal's retirement loomed in the minds of students, faculty, and parents, but no one was notified of the date of his retirement which had been scheduled and rescheduled many times. When the principal did retire in the summer, it was not publicly announced until September. There was much concern about the possibility of violence erupting in the fall session of the school. Part of the explosive tendency may have been related to anger and feelings of loss of the principal, revengeful wishes about his past rigid, repressive methods, as well as a displacement of these onto his replacement, coupled with fear of the stranger—the new principal.

Although the new principal had been a high school teacher, he was unknown to the present student body and his behavior and expectations in that role were unknown to students and teachers. Ruth Eissler (1949) noted that riots occurred in a delinquent girls' institution during the period of transition from very rigid discipline to a more liberal attitude. Thus there was an expectation, with forebodings of further disruption potentially during the fall. The PTA President and Vice President were perceptive and tried to prevent this from occurring by doing something positive before the school year began. Thus planning for the forum began before school opened and it was implemented several weeks after.

Eissler (1949) stated that:

> Whenever the equilibrium among the group of adults was labile, either because of changes in personnel or because of dissension within that group, although the children were not taken into their confidence, they reacted with rising tension . . . any change in the atmosphere of the adult's world which surrounded them constituted immediate danger and produced anxiety. . . . What seems to be incomprehensible, irrational behavior on the child's part, at closer investigation reveals itself as a mirror image of the grown-up's irrational behavior, an image produced by one of those mirrors which distort the original object. . . . If we compare the phenomenon of riot with the one of panic then we cannot avoid the conclusion that riots seem to have an integrating social function at least for their duration. Instead of complete isolation of the individual and disruption of object relations, as occurs in the case of panics, in riots identification of the individual group members with each other takes place on the basis of identical guilt feelings. . . . The riot is an emergency defense against the acute danger of panic.

When members of a family know their roles, have a balanced division of labor, are father-led but not dominated by father or mother, there is decreased adolescent pathology even when parents have psychopathology (Westley and Epstein, 1970). These factors provide a medium for homeostasis in the family. Thus, if there is the opposite input by the leaders' disequilibrium, adolescent psychopathology is more likely. Translating family for school, and parents for principal and faculty, conveys the meaningfulness of this percept to a broader field and supports Eissler's comments. The threat of downward and upward social mobility, mentioned earlier, to a sense of identity also has a bearing, then, on the potential for a riot, which was the case in this high school.

Ochberg and Trickett (1970), in studying the administrator's responses to racial conflict in a high school, noted that, "As long as social disruption is filtering down to the high school and junior high school, as long as high schools fail to provide institutionalized means of planning for change, the administrators of many schools will be saddled with responsibilities for which they are not particularly trained." The school they described was one in which there was a transition in the racial composition when redistricting of the school population changed the school's composition. It may also have had difficulty owing to the administrator of the school not functioning as an administrator, which contributed to the disequilibrium and development of the crisis in the youngsters.

Thus it is apparent that the teachers must also have been experiencing a good deal of disequilibrium in our high school, since they, particularly, were going to be exposed to a new principal who had formerly been a peer, and they did not know how he would treat them or function in his new role. His response was to tighten up and institute new rules to make sure that the previous trouble would not recur. This was the basis of the fears of the PTA officers, since this would have inevitably led to further rebellion, further restrictions by the principal, and an ever-inceasing circle of pressure and counterpressure leading like a crescendo to an explosion. It seems that this did not occur due to the forum leader's intervention and the positive results of the forum.

Rueveni (1971) developed a sensitivity group approach in a junior high school. He limited it to 15 aggressive students (out of a school population of 1500) who were characterized by their destructive, absentee and assaultive behavior, and with whom the teachers had been unable to cope. It was led by a white psychologist and co-led by a black woman counselor at the school. The students were selected from 30 names which the teachers submitted as likely candidates. Each student was asked if he wished to join the group; 20 accepted, but five dropped out within the first two weeks. This was apparently a very successful effort and was enlarged upon during the following year. However, in a way it limited itself to only the most troublesome students, but they had a choice of volunteering after they had been spotlighted.

In our arrangements there was no offer of a therapeutic contract. The contract was an offer to have an open forum, a dialogue, an opportunity to meet, ventilate, exchange feelings, and communicate. It was not limited, since it was available to all people connected with the school.

Others have used peers as resources in various therapy situations. Stone and Gilbert (1971) described the peer confrontation groups in a veterans' ward in which they used role modeling, systematic reassignments of members to groups, rotating more experienced group leaders, and each leader taking his turn as a "patient" to be confronted at every group session. This program seemed to be effective for these veterans using the peer confrontation method. Hilgard and associates (1969) have used better adjusted peers as models and leaders in group therapy with adolescents. Szymanski and Fleming (1971) arranged a therapeutic encounter in prison between a juvenile delinquent and an adult prisoner with some positive results accruing to a small number of inmates.

At our forum there certainly was peer confrontation, and the better adjusted students or adults came to the aid of other students or adults. For instance, when the most militant student became involved in an intense transference reaction to the forum chairman, a number of the students told him that he "had better lay off" and that he "better not start any trouble or they were going to get him." When one of the group leaders behaved like the adolescent by trying to thwart authority and undo understanding of the group process along with his own role as a group leader, many of the other adults and students did not side with him. They used their own values and some of those incorporated from the other adults, other group leaders, and the chairman of the forum.

Speck (1967) pioneered network therapy to deal with a crisis and avoid hospitalization for a potentially severe disorganization or suicidal attempt. He arranged a setting to try "to loosen the binds and tighten the bonds between people." This involved large group meetings whereby 75 to 100 or more people meet in someone's living room with the designated patient as the focal point initially, then moving out into the intergenerational and other areas of conflict in the large network with which the patient is involved. The additional support and effect of peers' information and interpretation in network therapy are important in handling the crisis (Sugar, 1971). There are both similarities and differences beteen network therapy and the forum: the forum was multigenerational as in Speck's (1967) vertical networks; there was no contract for therapy, which is in contrast to the network therapy arrangement where the contract is for therapy; there was no effort made at confidentiality and whatever was said in the group was not privileged communication to anyone present, as in network therapy.

Although there was no promise of confidentiality in the forum, to our knowledge none of the information given at the group sessions was used against the students by the parents, other students, or the teachers. Several of the students confessed to drug use, and their guilt feelings were the most important thing that emerged. They had to contend with themselves, although they expected the group leaders or parents to chastise them, or inform their parents or other authorities. There were references, but no confessions, to loose sexual standards and behavior, and this again was respected as information that was not to be used against the person relating it. The object of open communication with lessening of the binds between the interracial, intergenerational, and interauthority level groups was facilitated by this approach. The students were respected, listened to, and heard by the parents and faculty with mental health professionals' guidance and catalysis.

When attacked for inconsistent policies or rigid, restrictive rules, the principal had to make some rearrangements. When some of the transference "heat" shifted off the principal and was displaced to the chairman of the forum, it helped the principal regain some equilibrium and apply some of his more sensitive qualities to the role of administrator. The fact that he was able to attend the student event, engage in it, and be accepted by the students is some measure of his ability to alter his function and of the fact that the forum had made some contribution to the greater acceptance of the principal and authorities by the students, and perhaps vice versa. The group leaders, through the forum, gave the principal time to accommodate himself to the new position.

Some consideration should also be given to the teachers having found themselves in a less troublesome atmosphere. Perhaps their rather rapid disappearance from the forum was their signal of feeling less troubled than expected about the new principal and the possible eruption of violence. There were no attacks on the teachers and no invasions of their classes during this particular school year. They were able to teach. The students used the opportunity given them for controls and learning to better control themselves. The students complained of apathy in the latter months of the forum, but this seemed to be part of a more normal type of adolescent phenomenon (Winnicott, 1962).

Thus, given an opportunity, students, parents, teachers and faculty of a high school were able to meet in an open forum manner under some professional mental health guidance, where applied group process turned a critical and potentially explosive situation into one of some mutual increased self-esteem. The students came to identify with the group leaders and took over the function of improving communication between students and faculty. The group leaders provided a safety valve for the principal, with support, guided visibility, and interchange with the students, and a moratorium during which he was helped to obtain equilibrium to function more comfortably and suitably. It would appear that the forum approach may be of value in other similar situations.

In the three years since the forum ended, the high school has continued to have a modified forum in the PTA meetings attended by students, parents and teachers without any professionals leading it but modeled after the forum. During this time there have been no further crises. Simultaneously, other high schools in the same city have made headlines due to mass fighting between black and white students, strikes, walkouts, invasion of schools by outsiders and other critical or disruptive events.

It seems that our forum's influence was involved a year after our forum ended when, in 1972, the superintendent of the public school system in New Orleans directed the formation of a specially qualified team of individuals to deal directly with the rising problem of student unrest and the resulting campus disturbances. The primary purpose of the team—designated a Conflict Resolution Team—was to prevent such crisis situations by working to bring students, teachers, and parents together to discuss problems, and develop a forum to improve school conditions. The team was charged with the responsibility to develop ways to establish better communication and understanding of problems stemming, for the most part, from desegregation.

The Conflict Resolution Team concept grew out of a series of consulations with principals in whose schools where there were serious instances of student unrest during the fall and winter of the 1971-72 school year. These were the result of racial conflict and an upsurge of student activism. It was decided that a team of persons who could go into a school community, initiate dialogue with students, staff, parents, and community representatives, and try to effect understanding between them would be helpful in schools having conflicts and potential conflict situations.

Team members were selected because of their diversity (three men, one woman; two blacks, two whites), background, the disciplines (social work, teaching, psychology) they represented, their school and community experiences, as well as their competency in group dynamics.

Although some crises and headlines continue in two high schools, this team has effectively managed them in short order.

SUMMARY

In order to prevent the possible repetition of violent eruptions, such as a school strike, class disruptions, and assaults on teachers or students, a forum was offered to students, parents and faculty of a senior high school. The school was in a period of transition with a change of principal and of biracial composition.

For a total of eight sessions, over seven months, group process was used in large and small group meetings voluntarily attended by students, their parents, teachers, and faculty. A demand schedule was arranged which varied from weekly meetings initially to monthly meetings near the end of the academic year. No therapy was offered; neither history-taking, probing, nor interpretive work was done.

From an antagonistic, boiling group of students who were ready to attack the authority represented by the new principal, there emerged a marked displacement to the forum leader. Simultaneously, the student body became more calm and cooperative, while the principal became a likable, more humane, and acceptable figure. Progressively, the militancy seemed to abate, with improved communication between generations and races. Meetings became less frequent, with fewer in attendance. The principal, teachers and student body had regained their equilibrium. Adults became credible to students.

During the latter part of the year members of the student council, joined later by one faculty member, organized their own separate "rap" sessions. By the end of the school year interest in the forum had dissipated, and the forum ended. The school had no violence, disruptions, or problems of any greater degree than ten ordinary fist fights between students during the year and into the following year.

Details of the forum and modification of group process, dilution and spacing of sessions, as well as shared leadership to manage the transference and avoid becoming a therapy group, indicate the special needs of this situation and the efforts made to meet them. Particular considerations involved the prejudicial and transitional factors in the high school.

REFERENCES

ANSHIN, R. N. (1970). The role of a psychiatric consultant to a public high school in racial transition—Challenge and response. Presented at the American Orthopsychiatric Association meeting, 1970.

ANTHONY, E. J. (1970). The reaction of parents to adolescents and their behavior. In *Parenthood, Its Psychology and Psychopathology*. E. J. Anthony and T. Benedek, eds. pp. 307-324. Boston: Little, Brown.

BETTELHEIM, B., and JANOWITZ, M. (1964). *Social Change and Prejudice*. New York: Free Press of Glencoe.

EISSLER, R. S. (1949). Riots. *Psychoanal. Study Child*, 3/4:449-460.

HILGARD, J. R., STAIGHT, D. C., and MOORE, U. W. (1969). Better adjusted peers as resources in group therapy with adolescents. *Journal of Psychology*, 73:75-100.

LIPPITT, R., POLANSKY, N., REDL, F., and ROSEN, S. (1958). The dynamics of power: a field study of social influence in groups of children. In *Readings in Social Psychology*, E. E. Macoby, T. M. Newcomb and E. L. Hartley, eds. pp. 251-264. New York: Holt, Rinehart and Winston.

OCHBERG, F. M., and TRICKETT, E. (1970). Administrative responses to racial conflict in a high school. *Community Mental Health Journal*, 6:470-482.

RUEVENI, U. (1971). Using sensitivity training with junior high school students. *Children*, 18:69-72.

SCHNELL, R. D., PECKMAN, A., and MILFORD, R. (1970). Problem solving structure for a local high school in the Rio Hondo service area. Unpublished.

SCHRAG, P. (1971). The Ellsberg affair. *Saturday Review of Literature*, 54:34-39. Nov. 1.

SPECK, R. (1967). Psychotherapy of the social network of a schizophrenic family. *Family Process*, 6:208-214.

STONE, W. V., and GILBERT, R. (1971). Peer confrontation—What, why and whether. Presented at American Psychiatric Association meeting, 1971.

SUGAR, M. (1971). Network psychotherapy of an adolescent. *Adolescent Psychiatry*, 1:464-478.

SYZMANSKI, L., and FLEMING, A. (1971). Juvenile delinquent and an adult prisoner: A therapeutic encounter? *Journal of American Academy of Child Psychiatry*, 10:308-320.

WESTLEY, W. A. and EPSTEIN, N. B. (1970). *The Silent Majority*. San Francisco: Jossey Bass.

WINNICOTT, D. W. (1962). Adolescence. *New Era in Home and School*, 43:1-7.

Part II
FAMILY THERAPY

9

Indications and Contraindications for Family Therapy

DANIEL OFFER, M.D. *and*
EVERT VANDERSTOEP, M.D.

INTRODUCTION

The purpose of this chapter is to outline the indications and contra-indications for family therapy. We will review the relevant literature and share our own clinical experiences in treating families. We are limiting ourselves to the treatment of families where there are two generations present. Our main interest is in families where one generation is represented by adolescents (puberty to the end of high school) and the other generation is composed of the parents of these children.

A number of family therapists have written on the subject of indications and contraindications for family therapy. These writings will be reviewed below. Significantly, a number of family therapists have *not* written on the subject of indications and contraindications for family therapy. These authors indicate that they believe that the question of indications and contraindications is a "non-question."

In order to condense a great deal of complex material one needs to develop a classification system. Practitioners of family therapy have been classified by Haley (1962), Haley and Hoffman (1968), and Beels et al. (1969). We developed yet another classification, based upon the examination of the literature on indications and contraindications for family therapy. Two distinct schools of thought emerge from the literature. These schools are: 1) the psychoanalysts; 2) the system analysts. This classification may be useful in trying to understand the fundamental theoretical struggle in the field of family therapy.

The Psychoanalysts

The following family therapists are selected to represent the psychoanalytic point of view: Ackerman (1966), Jackson (1959), Kramer (1970), Wynne (1965), and Williams (1967). They hold to a nosological psychiatric classification system and conceptualize individuals and families along psychodynamic and psychopathologic points of view. For them, doing a diagnostic family interview enables the psychotherapist to diagnose psychopathological processes and thus arrive at both the family and individual diagnoses. With a diagnosis at hand, one can then select the most appropriate treatment or group of treatments. The nosological psychopathological point of view is very natural to the practitioners in the field of family therapy who are physicians. It employs the standard medical notion: disease—investigate—arrive at a diagnosis—select a proper treatment. There are very few non-physicians in the field of family therapy who belong to this group.

For Jackson (1959), family interviewing is superior to collaborative work. More relevant data are gathered in family interviews which enable the therapist to arrive at a better diagnosis. He distinguishes among four categories of families: (1) stable satisfactory; (2) unstable satisfactory; (3) unstable unsatisfactory; and (4) stable unsatisfactory.

Families of the first category do not need therapy. He finds the unstable satisfactory category one in which the best results are obtained from family therapy. In these families there is usually enough mutual regard between the spouses for the therapist to intervene directly. These people married because they were in love and usually still are in love. The unstable unsatisfactory family comprises the largest bulk of severe psychopathology. In these families the nominal patient's recovery often poses a serious threat to the parents. There is only limited success in treating these families.

Finally, in families of the stable unsatisfactory category, Jackson reports poor results. In a brief case report, he describes a family session in which the nominal patient's brother, emboldened by his relationship to the therapist, tentatively offered some comments critical of his mother. The following morning, the mother was taken to the hospital for an emergency cholecystectomy, and upon her return from the hospital, the father was hospitalized for a coronary heart attack and, in the midst of all this, the brother had an automobile accident in which he crashed into the rear of the car ahead. The family at this point decided they could no longer afford family therapy and placed the patient in a state hospital. Jackson's view was that treatment of the stable unsatisfactory family is a very risky undertaking.

Wynne (1965) states that he considers family therapy the treatment of choice under certain conditions. He feels that there are certain limitations which are intrinsic to family therapy and other limitations are imposed by external practical conditions. For exploratory family therapy a stable structured treatment setup is essential. An implied contraindication to family therapy is a situation in which a stable structured treatment setup is not possible. Family diagnosis—a necessary precursor to exploratory family therapy—may include home visits, psychological testing and interviews with individual family members, and does not require a stable treatment structure. Family diagnosis is for the purpose of formulating a well considered strategy.

The general indications for exploratory family therapy, according to Wynne, are a need for clarification and resolution of intrafamilial difficulties. In addition, family therapy provides a preferable approach to individual psychoanalytic or psychodynamic psychotherapies when a transference relationship cannot be established. Ideally, all family members should have a vital and continuing stake in the treatment. In order to set the stage for future possible family therapy, conjoint sessions are a necessary part of the initial evaluation.

Wynne lists a number of psychiatric problems for which exploratory family therapy seems best suited:

(1) Adolescents' separation problems. The diagnostic problem here is whether the chief issue is an identity crisis or rebellious delinquent behavior. The problem is defined as an individual one if an identity conflict exists in the adolescent. However, for those adolescents who failed to emerge from a symbiotic dependency relationship with a parent, exploratory family therapy is indicated.

(2) The trading of dissociations. This involves an intricate network of perceptions about other family members and dissociations about one's own qualities. In this situation each family member projects a particular quality or feeling onto another family member.

(3) Collective cognitive chaos and erratic distancing. These are families with schizophrenic members who manifest bizarre, disruptive threats and episodes. The members of these families suffer from a shared sense of being unable to reach one another on any feeling level. Each family member is painfully aware of his own need and wishes for relatedness but each feels that the

others block intimacy. Some of the shared mechanisms for maintaining these exclusions have been described by Wynne under the headings of pseudomutuality and pseudohostility.

(4) Amorphous communication. These families, mostly with a schizophrenic member, have an amorphous, vague and distorted form of communication.

An important ingredient in family therapy is the skill of the therapist. Wynne discusses several areas of skills that must be attained before one becomes a competent family therapist. By implication then, he maintains that family therapy is contraindicated when a skilled family therapist is not available.

Kramer (1970) provides a descriptive list of indications and contraindications for family therapy. As is true of the other writers mentioned here, these ideas are gained from clinical and supervisory experience and hence must be recognized to be impressionistic.

He theorizes that there are two sets of problems: (1) the intrapsychic; and (2) the interpersonal. One can distinguish between these two types of problems—often just on the basis of the way the problem is presented to the therapist on the telephone.

When the problem is presented as a difficulty the family is having with a certain member, or when the complaint is about trouble a family member is having with society, it is most likely an interpersonal problem, and family therapy will be indicated. If the problem is presented in terms such as the unhappiness, shyness, or low self-esteem of a family member, the problem is likely to be intrapsychic, and individual therapy will be indicated. However, Kramer would recommend in any case that evaluation be done with the family rather than with an individual for several reasons. The first, of course, is to evaluate thoroughly if the problem is primarily intrapsychic or interpersonal and decide if family therapy is the treatment of choice. In addition, family evaluation provides a preparation for family interviews should they become necessary during the course of an individual treatment. Yet another important use of a series of family interviews would be preparation for psychoanalysis: "The structuralizing and synthesizing effect of successful family therapy converts acting-out aspects of a character disorder into an internalized neurosis."

Kramer also believes family therapy to be markedly more successful in helping families manage the care of a severely ill member—physically or psychiatrically—than individual treatment.

A complete list of Kramer's indications and contraindications will be found in Table I.

Shapiro (1967) stresses the importance of delineation, by which he means the image one person has of another. When these delineations are markedly inconsistent, exaggerated and destructive in nature, family therapy is indicated in order to correct the family members' view of each other. "The family session is an excellent situation in which to establish the actuality of the adolescent's maturation in the idiosyncratic and defensive aspects of the parents' response to it."

Howells (1972) believes that a family orientation is a necessary background for all therapies. However, he has found family therapy unsuccessful and hence contraindicated in families with a member who suffers from "process schizophrenia." This diagnostic entity is more clearly defined in Europe than in the United States. Investigators like Friedman and his associates (1965), Lidz, Fleck and Cornelison (1965) and Wynne (1965) would probably disagree with Howells's statement.

Ackerman (1966) believes that family therapy should promote a sense of well-being, getting rid of something a person is suffering from. But it is not enough to expunge the bad without being prepared to replace it with something better. Unless the patient is able to envision a new and better way of living, he will cling to his old way. Families at any one time exhibit both health-maintaining forces and health-eroding forces. The balance shifts with time and the vicissitudes of life situations. Wellness and sickness are value concepts that reflect a way of life.

When a conflict cannot be adequately contained, it spills over into irrational acting out. On other occasions the control of the conflict fails, leading to progressive disorganization in family relations. Prejudicial scapegoating is a result of conflicts being misperceived and hence, uncontained and unresolved.

In evaluating families, Ackerman stresses that we must keep in mind the goals of psychotherapy. They are to remove disabling symptoms, to strengthen the patient's personality, to enable the person to realize his potential by capitalizing on his resources, and to help the patient become an efficient, productive and happy human being. The method is influenced by many factors: (1) personal expectations of the patient; (2) orientation of the psychotherapist towards his role; (3) group influences surrounding the patient; and (4) group influences surrounding the therapist.

Family therapy can appropriately be applied to a wide range of behavior disorders. It can be useful in the treatment of neurosis, psychosis and character disorders, especially those that show acting out, but it must be flexibly accommodated to the specific and unique features of each of these conditions. It is especially helpful in those conditions in which the here-and-now struggle with interpersonal conflicts of the family potentially affects the outcome of coping with intrapsychic conflicts. Family therapy is also uniquely effective with marital disorders and with disturbances involving the relationship of children and adolescents with the family.

TABLE I

INDICATIONS AND CONTRAINDICATIONS FOR FAMILY THERAPY

INDICATIONS	CONTRAINDICATIONS
Jackson:	
Unstable-Satisfactory	
Unstable-Unsatisfactory	Stable-Unsatisfactory
Wynne:	
Adolescent separation problems	Some severe depressions
Trading dissociations	Some severe masochistic states
Collective cognitive chaos and erratic distancing	Acute schizophrenia
Fixed distancing with eruptive threats and episodes	Lack of structured treatment setting
Amorphous communication	Unavailability of skilled family therapist
Kramer:	
Majority of complaints interpersonal	Some therapist converting from individual to family therapy
Conflict between family members and society	A firm decision to divorce
Acute family crisis	Severe psychotic depression
Families with poorly structured ego and chronically disturbed functioning	Hard core psychopathy
	Severe masochistic character
Unsuccessful individual treatment	Chronic schizophrenic psychosis
Supervision of one family member	One family member in intensive individual treatment
Learning blocks in children	An older adolescent who is preoccupied with disengagement from the family
Preparation for psychoanalysis	
Shapiro:	
Markedly inconsistent images held by parents and the adolescent of each other	
Howells:	
Necessary background for all therapies	Process schizophrenia

INDICATIONS

Whitaker:

Necessary background for all therapies

Ackerman:

A wide range of behavior disorders, especially:
 (1) interpersonal conflicts that effect outcome of intrapsychic conflicts
 (2) reducing secondary gains of emotional illness
 (3) marital disturbances
 (4) disturbances with relationship of children and adolescents
 (5) acting out (delinquency, drug abuse, sexual promiscuity)

CONTRAINDICATIONS

Unskilled family therapist
Severe psychosomatic illness

The process of a malignant, irreversible trend toward breakup of the family, which may mean that it is too late to reverse the process of fragmentation
The dominance within the group of a concentrated focus of malignant, destructive motivation
One parent who is afflicted with an organized progressive paranoid condition, or with incorrigible psychopathic destructiveness or who is a confirmed criminal or pervert
Parents, one or both, who are unable to be sufficiently honest; lying and deceitfulness that are deeply rooted in the group negate the potential usefulness of family therapy
The existence of a certain kind of valid family secret
The existence of an unyielding cultural, religious, or economic prejudice against this form of intervention
The existence in some members of extremely rigid defenses which, if broken, might induce a psychosis, a psychosomatic crisis or physical assault
Finally, the presence of organic disease or other disability of a progressive nature that precludes the participation of one or more members.

The System Analysts

The non-medical practitioners in the field of family therapy may experience the medically oriented disease-treatment scheme as foreign to them. The system analysts are practitioners who view people in distress as part of a system and believe that nosology and psychopathology are potential interferences with the most helpful response. Such a response can only occur when the two systems engage each other in a most open and flexible way.

Unterberger (1972) believes that discussion of when to do and not to do family therapy can be an externalization of the therapist's question of himself: "What am I willing to do and what do I not want to do?" To say that a family is unfit for family therapy because they are unmotivated may mean that they would not come to the office. Then home visits are in order. To say that the inability to convene a full family session is a contraindication may miss critical issues for that family. When a therapist takes the time and energy to convene the family network, a considerable amount of therapeutic work is accomplished in that process. Sharing clear statements about what we want to accomplish with a family with those involved often paves the way to effective interventions with "untreatable" families.

In the system analysts' view, everyone—therapists and patients alike—is limited by the developmental level of his current systems. Good therapy takes place when patients are fortunate enough to encounter a system with which they can accomplish mutual growth. Hence, all concerns about disease and psychopathology become irrelevant. The only important thing is the potential for mutual evolution and change in the two intermeshing systems.

A well-known expositor of this view is Whitaker (in Haley and Hoffman, 1968). A good deal of the thrust of Whitaker's work can be described by the term "the growing edge" (Whitaker, as quoted by Haley and Hoffman, 1968). He believes that the most crucial factor in indications for family therapy is the presence of a skilled family therapist. A great deal of respect for the power of the two generation systems has prompted Whitaker to insist that family therapy be done by two therapists. Briefly, co-therapy is only possible where the therapists respect each other. And as most system analysts and psychoanalysts maintain, one should never schedule interviews at the outset of treatment with less than the entire family in attendance.

Haley (1971a) has some strong words to say on the matter of indications and contraindications for family therapy. He clearly states that he believes it is a "non-question." He states that the more experienced family therapist will appear puzzled since he finds defining any kind of therapy as a way of intervening with a family. Psychopathology is redefined as a relationship problem and the unit of diagnosis and treatment is no longer the individual but is the family.

Explorations of the genetic background of unsatisfactory patterns can be safely dispensed with, since they are a bore to the patients and a waste of time. Psychodynamics may be interesting to the therapist but are not useful to people in distress. Understanding of one's interpersonal operations is not helpful because what is needed is *change* and understanding does not produce change. Different interpersonal operations with their own feedback and redundancies must be established for therapy to take place. The agent of change is change itself.

Haley (1971b) discusses contraindications for family therapy when he describes the disquieting effect upon the standard outpatient clinic of the introduction of family therapy methods. Several reasons are advanced for this disquieting effect. The usual existing hierarchy will be disrupted inasmuch as most staff members will be students in family therapy and hence, the old division of who does and knows more than whom will be completely changed. This can develop to the point where the lower pay scale professional staff are more skilled than the higher pay scale staff.

The other disquieting aspect of the introduction of family therapy methods is that it requires the abandonment of highly cherished theoretical systems and requires that they be replaced by the interpersonal theories. Also, the emphasis on diagnosis and evaluation, which, according to Haley, is a device to deal with the therapist's anxiety, has to be replaced with an action oriented point of view, in which experienced therapists share an awareness that much can be accomplished with active intervention. The primary concern in evaluation becomes how the family responds to intervention by that particular therapist or co-therapy team. When a family meets the therapist, their systems are interacting and progress is a product of these interactions.

McGregor (1972) states that family therapy is indicated when the family can be convened and it is not indicated when the family cannot be convened.

The system analysts do believe that many helpful forces can be brought to bear on the family system in distress. Such methods as behavioral modification techniques, individual psychotherapies and group psychotherapies all find their place in a natural evolution from the base of the naturally occurring system—the family.

In summary, the system analysts regard discussion of indications and contraindications as not meaningful and not germane to principal therapy issues. For them the only possible approach to distress is attending to the systems. The system that will most probably receive attention is the family system.

THE FAMILY IN PSYCHOTHERAPY

Psychotherapeutic interventions involving the family as a system are of recent origin. Freud early recognized that the relationship between the generations is of utmost importance for the mental health of the child. In the case of little Hans (1909) he treated the child through his father, although he did not see the child himself. Later, in the child guidance movement in America the team approach was instituted where a family was treated in the clinic, but never together in the same room. The child had his own therapist as did the parents.

It was not until shortly after World War II that investigators began seeing the family as a psychosocial unit with its own aims, problems, psychopathology and coping devices. It was felt then that if the unit was treated *together* at the same time and by the same therapist, the changes which would take place through therapy would affect the family as a whole. Thus, if the family changed its styles of adaptation and the nature of the relationship between its members, a new homeostasis would develop. Roles would change and an opportunity for new experiences would take place. The stereotyped and rigid relationships between the generations would be lessened and hence a potential for growth through learning would arise. Open and flowing communication was seen as an essential ingredient for the functioning of a relatively healthy family.

We do not intend in this article to explore the difficult question of what are the characteristics of a normal or healthy family. For physicians in general, and psychiatrists in particular, it is easier to describe the characteristics of a disturbed family. For purposes of this article a disturbed family is defined as one which has come to the psychotherapist and asked for help. The family can be self-referred or referred by a friend or another professional. They can have a nominal patient, often defined as the "scapegoat" (see Bell and Vogel, 1960), or they can feel that they have a family problem.

It often happens that relatively new psychotherapeutic techniques develop "schools" or become "movements." The adherents of the new school extol the virtues of the technique, find its leaders charismatic and have the tendency to dump other forms of treatment. This overreaction to the appearance of a perfectly valid new technique has the tendency to: (1) make enemies of the adherents to the old schools who have not tried the new method but are suspicious because of the excessive claims made by disciples of the new school; (2) cause the practitioners of the new school to overextend themselves and try to cure all mental illnesses with their new "cure-all" approach; and (3) lead to inevitable disappointments in patients and psychotherapists alike.

We believe that the field of family therapy has reached the stage where we can begin to take a sober look at both the achievements and the failures of this particular approach. We have chosen family therapy with adolescents because this is a period during the life span of the individual when intergenerational conflicts are expected to arise. Consequently, it might be helpful to work with the total family when an adolescent is involved; such family therapy does, however, also create special problems.

It has been our experience that, in general, we can divide adolescents into four groups (regardless of their diagnosis):

1. *The Individual*—The adolescent who states emphatically that he has a personal problem for which he seeks help and under no circumstances does he want to be in a room with his parents.

2. *The Individual as Part of the Family*—The adolescent who states that he will come into treatment only if his whole family comes because there is a family problem.

3. *The Individual as Part of the Group*—Lately we have seen a number of adolescents who claim to have peer-group problems. They want to be treated only in group therapy.

4. *The Large Group of Adolescents Who Fall in the Continuum Between Groups 1, 2, and 3.*

The parents can, of course, also be divided similarly into four groups. The above groups do not necessarily correspond to those who, theoretically, we believe could benefit from family therapy. It is important to stress that the therapist should take into account the initial bias that the patient brings with him. A charismatic therapist can often convince the patient to try another approach, depending on how deep the conviction is in the patient.

At times the specific belief system or cultural environment precludes the use of family therapy. For example, one of us has recently seen a 15-year-old acting-out adolescent girl for evaluation. There was much discontent among the parents: the mother was depressed and the father readily admitted to having extramarital affairs. The girl had run away from home on numerous occasions, had acted out sexually, was angry and did poorly in school. She readily admitted that she needed psychotherapy. She absolutely refused to be seen together with her parents. One of her parents underwent psychoanalytic treatment some years back and all her friends in the private high school where she was a student told her that she had to have "transference" to her psychotherapist and only through this would she be helped. Here the therapist has a relatively simple choice: he can begin seeing her in individual psychotherapy or refer her to another therapist.

We would like to stress another form of distortion which often may affect the therapist. In a particular community a therapist begins to be known for his expertise in working with a particular set of problems or special kind of patients. If his field is family therapy, he would tend to get referrals from colleagues, other mental health professionals and former patients which coincide with his major interest. The initial screening has already been done for him. When he meets with the family for an evaluation he finds that more often than not they belong to the second group of patients—those who want to work as a family. In the past five years over 60% of the adolescents between the ages of 13 and 17 who were referred to us by colleagues or other mental health professionals came specifically for family therapy.

One might get the erroneous impression that most adolescents are amenable or interested in family therapy. This is not the case. One of us recently moved his private office to a new location where his interests in family therapy were not known. The first four teenagers that he saw have all had family therapy in the past and stated that under no circumstances would they try it again!

It is obvious from the short discussion above that we do not believe that there is one type of psychotherapeutic technique which is applicable to most adolescent problems. There are many variables which have to be considered, including the value system of the patients. For the relatively healthy adolescent most psychotherapeutic methods used by an expert will prove helpful. For the very disturbed, most psychotherapeutic techniques are inadequate. A firmly developed therapeutic alliance based on positive initial impression (likability factor) is often more important than the type of intervention used.

We would disagree with those who say that failure to convene the family is a function of the therapist's lack of commitment to family therapy. At times failure to convene a family may indeed indicate a problem in the therapist's commitment. However, the following case vignette is offered to illustrate that family therapy is not always possible even when it is clearly indicated. In this case, to be effective, we had to operate as Bowen (1966) has suggested—by treating the family through one member.

The therapist met this patient when she was 18 years of age. She had had a series of therapists and therapeutic encounters, including an experience with family therapy. In each case, the therapy was aborted either because the therapist couldn't stand the patient or the patient couldn't stand the therapist. However, she liked the present therapist from the beginning, and the therapist liked her, though he found her very trying. After struggling alone with her and her parents for six months in separate meetings, the therapist recognized that he needed help and introduced a co-therapist. No amount of documentation of the complementarity of the family members' moods and behavior could persuade this family to meet as a family. The therapist did browbeat the parents into agreeing to meet with the patient and the therapists every third week and they did so for 18 months; however, the only recorded effect of such interviews was that the parents fought more for a few days following each interview. The interviews with the parents did provide the therapists with a backlog of experience and enabled them to speak with the daughter about her parents from a position of experience.

Over several years of treatment, the strong symbiotic tie between mother and daughter and the strong support that the father gave to his daughter so that she would be able to tolerate a life of sacrificing everything to her mother have gradually been unraveled and loosened. The process of treatment so far has been very encouraging in that serious suicide attempts are a thing of the past and the daughter has been able to achieve a measure of calm and some satisfaction and joy in her life. She has not as yet achieved independence from her parents.

The above demonstrates that therapists need to be flexible and work with a family when feasible and appropriate but not withdraw when one part of the system refuses to go on. The family may not always cooperate with family therapy. This might be particularly true if the parents are threatened by the potential improvement in their child without seeing any benefits in it for them. Although family interviews were contraindicated in this case, the family was treated in absentia.

It is very important to select the functional social subsystem for participation in family therapy. And it should be clear that this functional social subsystem may, but does not necessarily, correspond to the legal definition of family. The unavailability of one or more members of a defined functional social subsystem may well be a contraindication to family therapy.

A necessary condition for exploratory family therapy is the stability of the membership that meets with the therapists. A further essential consideration when making a recommendation for family therapy is the phase in the psychotherapeutic process. There may come a time in exploratory family therapy when individual therapy should supplant the family therapy, or it may be that family therapy would be contraindicated initially if intrapsychic problems were prominent and needed to be dealt with at the outset. Some depressed or severely masochistic individuals, who soak up all the blame for the family difficulties, need a period of individual therapy before family therapy can get off the ground.

In families with an acutely schizophrenic member who is still in panic and has not yet established a relationship with a therapist, family therapy is contraindicated. Such patients may not be able to tolerate the complexities of family interviews. In these situations, it may be best to delay family interviews for a month or two until the psychotic individual has developed some trust in the therapist and the panic has diminished.

There are a number of psychological routes from childhood to adulthood. One type of normal middle-class suburban adolescent goes through adolescence with relatively few overt conflicts (Offer, 1969). His behavior, in general, does not conflict with parental values and his rebellion, which occurs in early adolescence, is in the service of emancipation and separation from the parents.

The disturbed adolescent may have a variety of psychodynamics which stem from different intrapsychic conflicts. There is nothing, however, which disturbs parents, teachers, law enforcement officers and society in general as much as an acting-out adolescent. The behavior of the acting-out adolescent may include promiscuity, drug abuse, delinquency, perversion, vandalism or violent behavior. These adolescents are seen as spiteful, angry, negativistic, solemn, narcissistic, egotistic and unconcerned with their fellowman. At times they have enough insight to know that they have problems. They often want help but find it hard to ward off impulses when they are together with their peers.

It is for these adolescents that family therapy can be particularly helpful. It shows the teenager and his family (parents and siblings) that the acting out has meaning. It is not performed in isolation. Rather, it often responds to verbal and nonverbal cues from other members of the family. In family therapy it is clearly demonstrated that the behavioral response on the part of one of the teenagers reflects tension in the whole family system. When the acting-out behavior stops, other parts of the family must show overt conflict; for example, the marital disharmony between father and mother does not come up to the surface until the acting out of their adolescent child has stopped. Even more dramatically the parents, together or separately, stimulate the acting out of their child in order to have an external problem to deal with. In our experience, acting-out behavior can be stopped most dramatically in family therapy.

Recently, one of us saw a 15-year-old boy who was referred because he was having behavior problems in the home and in school and because there was active sexual play between him and his eight-year-old sister.

The parents had a poor relationship. The boy did not want psychotherapy. Only after a number of family sessions, where it was pointed out to the entire family that they had a "family problem," did the boy consent to come for help. It was not long before the family realized that there was considerable similarity between the boy's acting out, the mother's seductive behavior and the father's solemn, depressed and withdrawn attitude. Symptom relief came relatively quickly (after three months). The tension in the family was reduced and the family was able to function on a higher level of integration. When communication was improved, understanding between the generations became possible.

SUMMARY

We have reviewed the relevant literature on the indications and contraindications for family therapy. We have divided the practitioners into two major groups: the psychoanalysts and the system analysts. Their points of view, their practical approaches and their recommendations have been discussed. We have also discussed our own clinical experience in treating families, stressing our belief that careful consideration must be given to the choice of therapy. Finally, we have outlined the conditions for which we believe family therapy to be the treatment of choice.

REFERENCES

ACKERMAN, N. W. (1966). *Treating the Troubled Family*. New York: Basic Books.

BEELS, C. C. ,and FERBER, A. (1969). Family therapy: A view. *Family Process*, Vol. 8, No. 2, September. Pp. 280-332. Comments by James L. Framo, F. Gentry Harris, Lyman C. Wynne, Gerald H. Zuk.

BELL, N. W., and VOGEL, E. F. (1960). The emotionally disturbed child as the family scapegoat. In *The Family*, N. W. Bell and E. F. Vogel, eds. Glencoe, Ill.: The Free Press.

BOWEN, M. (1966). The use of family theory in clinical practice. *Comprehensive Psychiatry*, 7:345-374.

FREUD, S. (1909). Analysis of a phobia in a five-year-old boy. *The Standard Edition of the Complete Psychological Works of S. Freud*, Vol. X. London: The Hogarth Press, 1955.

FRIEDMAN, A. S., BOSZORMENYI-NAGY, I., JUNGREIS, J. E., LINCOLN, G., MITCHELL, H. E., SONNE, J. C., SPECK, R. V., SPIVACK, G. (1965). *Psychotherapy for the Whole Family*. New York: Springer Publishing Company, Inc.

HALEY, J. (1962). Whither family therapy. *Family Process*, 1:69-100.

HALEY, J., and HOFFMAN, L. (1968). An interview with Carl A. Whitaker. In *Techniques of Family Therapy*. J. Haley and L. Hoffman, eds. Pp. 473-480. New York: Basic Books.

HALEY, J. (1971a). Family therapy. *International Journal of Psychiatry*, 9:233-242.

HALEY, J. (1971b). Why a mental health clinic should avoid family therapy. Manuscript, Philadelphia.

HOWELLS, J. G. (1972). Personal communication.

JACKSON, D. (1959). Family interaction, family homeostasis and implication for therapy. In *Individual and Family Dynamics,* J. Masserman, ed. New York: Grune and Stratton.

KRAMER, C. H. (1970). Psychoanalytically oriented family therapy: Ten year evolution in a private child psychiatry practice. Family Institute of Chicago Publication. No. 1. Pp. 1-42.

LIDZ, T., FLECK, S., and CORNELISON, A. (1965). *Schizophrenia and the Family.* New York: International Universities Press.

McGREGOR, R. (1972). Personal communication.

OFFER, D. (1969). *The Psychological World of the Teen-Ager.* New York: Basic Books.

SHAPIRO, R. L. (1967). The origin of adolescent disturbances in the family: Some considerations in therapy and implications for therapy. In *Family Therapy and Disturbed Families,* G. H. Zuk and I. Boszormenyi-Nagy, eds. Palo Alto: Science and Behavior Books.

UNTERBERGER, L. (1972). Personal communication.

WHITAKER, C. A. (1972). Personal communication.

WILLIAMS, F. S. (1967). Family therapy: A critical assessment. *American Journal of Orthopsychiatry,* October, 37:912-919.

WYNNE, L. C. (1965). Some indications and contraindications for exploratory family therapy. In *Intensive Family Therapy: Theoretical and Practical Aspects,* I. Boszormenyi-Nagy and J. L. Framo, eds. Pp. 289-322. New York: Harper and Row.

10

Countertransference in Family Therapy with Adolescents

Helm Stierlin, M.D., Ph.D.

"Countertransference" in family therapy refers to phenomena that are controversial, ambiguous and complex. To unravel this ambiguity and complexity we must, at first, briefly trace the shifting and widening meanings of the terms "transference" and "countertransference" in psychoanalytic therapy.

TRANSFERENCE IN THE PSYCHOANALYTIC SITUATION

Freud mentioned the term "transference" for the first time in 1895 in his *Studies in Hysteria*. He defined it in 1905, when publishing the Dora case, as a "special class of mental structures, for the most part unconscious. . . ." These are "new editions or facsimiles of the impulses and fantasies which are aroused and made conscious during the progress of analysis; but they have this peculiarity, which is characteristic for their species, that they replace some earlier person by the person of the physician" (p. 116).

After this definition was made, Freud and his followers widened our perspective on transference. They described its affective and perceptual components, distinguished between positive, negative, and ambivalent transferences, and related these to the dynamics of introjection, projection, repression, and acting out (e.g., the view was held that memories which are repressed and cannot be remembered must be repetitively acted out as transferences). Also, they developed the concept of the transference neurosis.

Transference phenomena—like Sullivan's parataxic distortions—were seen as ubiquitous. However, they were held to have special affinity to the psychoanalytic situation. It was this situation which bred them in pure culture, as it were, and which also provided optimal conditions for their examination and final resolution. The patient as well as the analyst structured this situation by sticking to the terms of the analytic contract: the patient mainly by trying to comply with the basic analytic rule (to say everything that came to his mind); the analyst chiefly by being "abstinent"—i.e., frustrating to the patient—but also stable, firm, and free from "blind spots." In his frustrating firmness, he became a bulwark against which the patient's transference processes could "bump," thus revealing their intensity and inappropriateness; in remaining free from blind spots, i.e., free from unconscious biases and neurotic anxieties, he could examine the patient's transference distortions empathically as well as objectively.

Inevitably, the above meaning of transference changed with the changing psychoanalytic situation. This happened when analysts began to analyze patients whom they had previously considered to be unanalyzable —such as schizophrenics, whom Freud had viewed as incapable of developing transference. The notion of the therapist as an abstinent, detached observer now became problematical and new aspects of transference came into focus. I have traced some of these in my book, *Conflict and Reconciliation* (1969), which deals with the special therapeutic situation required for schizophrenic patients.

COUNTERTRANSFERENCE IN THE PSYCHOANALYTIC SITUATION

Countertransference can be viewed as the mirror concept of transference. Freud introduced it in 1910 in his paper on the future prospects of psychoanalytic therapy. Almost from this time on, the term "countertransference," even more than transference, has remained ambiguous and controversial.

Essentially, two major meanings emerged: first, countertransference was viewed simply as the analyst's reaction to the patient's transference; and, second, it was defined as the analyst's transference to the patient for other reasons. These differing meanings then created different vantage points for further observations and conceptualizations. Within the first definition, countertransference primarily provided information about the patient. The therapist used his own feelings and reactions as major data about the patient. Within the second definition, the therapist tended to emerge as a stumbling block to his patient's progress. The focus was now on his blind spots, neurotic or character problems, rigidities, etc., which interfered with his patient's unfolding transference, therapeutic progress, and growth.

Often these two aspects—the information-providing aspect and the stumbling block aspect—are interwoven, as when a (usually mild) stumbling block in the therapist also facilitates pertinent information about a certain patient. M. B. Cohen (1952) has well illustrated such clinical situations. Since such interactions between the two meanings occur frequently, I shall not here make a deliberate choice between them.

As happened with transference phenomena, processes of countertransference became more difficult to assess as the classic, dyadic analytic situation with a well-motivated, neurotic patient became less prevalent. The contributions of H. Searles (1959), F. Fromm-Reichmann (1950), D. W. Winnicott (1958), and others on countertransference in the treatment of schizophrenics are here illuminating. Searles used his countertransference reactions chiefly as primary data sources on the complex dynamics of his schizophrenic patients. For example, he described *his* (the therapist's) own vengefulness, primitive wishes for fusion, feared loss of boundaries, etc. as signals alerting him to corresponding or complementary experiences in his patients. F. Fromm-Reichmann and D. W. Winnicott, in contrast, focused rather on those personality aspects or "blind spots" in the therapists of schizophrenics—such as an excessive conventionality, or use of intellectualization as defense—which could seriously limit their therapeutic effectiveness.

TRANSFERENCE AND COUNTERTRANSFERENCE IN GROUPS

Groups introduce new therapeutic and conceptual paradigms and added complexities. Even more than in dyadic relations, the terms transference and countertransference become problematical here. Although a group consists of individual patients with individual problems, we must now focus on the whole multi-person unit, and, where applicable, conceive of the group as *the* patient. Freud (1921), Bion (1961), Ezriel (1950), and many others have described typical group dynamics.

Transference and countertransference phenomena (or their analogues) in groups, like those occurring in individual therapy, are shaped by the patients' and therapist's contributions to the therapeutic situation. The special quality of the patients' contributions derives mainly from the fact that they constitute an "ad hoc" group, i.e., an aggregate of people who lack a common history, real life bonds and commitments to each other beyond those resulting from their transient group experience. Within such an ad hoc group, typical group processes and group fantasies can unfold. The group therapist or leader, who follows a psychoanalytic model and remains abstinent, influences on his part these group processes and fantasies.

Bion (1961), Turquet (1965, 1971) Argelander (1972), and others have described the leader's contributions chiefly to those group fantasies which unfold in small groups, also called Bion groups. The leader of such groups must be abstinent to an unusual degree. Thereby, he structures and maintains an "asymmetry" between himself and the group. By avoiding all acting out with the group and by giving interpretations on the group level only, he insures that the group stews in its own anxiety, as it were. In this way, the group members are forced to rely on their own resources, i.e., to seek and find largely their own answers to emerging problems.

In addition to reflecting the differing contributions of patients and therapists, the concepts of transference and countertransference have come to reveal the differing theoretical leanings (e.g., more Freudian or Kleinian) of group therapists. Grotjahn (1953), for example, standing mainly in the classical psychoanalytic tradition, has distinguished three major transference dynamics in groups: first, the transference relation to the therapist—or central figure—presumably developing out of a transference neurosis, as patterned in psychoanalysis; second, the transference relation between the members of the group to each other; and, third, a transference developed to the group as a pre-oedipal mother.

My own view on transference and countertransference in groups builds essentially on the ideas of Bion and the Tavistock group as represented, among others, by Turquet (1965, 1971), Rice (1969), Shapiro and Zinner (in press), and Rioch (1971).

Group transference and countertransference processes, according to this view, interlock with the vicissitudes of certain typical group fantasies. These group fantasies mirror, as well as shape, certain types of recurrent group behavior. At the same time, they give evidence of characteristic "basic assumptions" which are shared by the whole group. Essentially, these are the basic assumptions of "dependence," "fight-flight," and "pairing," as originally described by Bion. They reflect, as well as derive from, a group climate which exerts a strong regressive pull. The members' shared sense of omnipotence, even while they lack a sense of responsibility and a sense for temporal sequences and realistic constraints, is here the most striking feature. It colors all fantasies that evolve, which often have a volatile, primary process quality.

These group fantasies—or basic assumptions—in turn structure the group's attitude toward, and perceptions and expectations of, the leader. Such group attitude we may then call the "group transference." The leader might either be approached and perceived as an all-giving and all-knowing super-father or -mother, able—though often not willing— to satisfy the exorbitant, regressive dependency needs of the group, or he may be perceived as an intrusive enemy whom the group must either fight or flee, or he might be perceived as a partner for, or enabler of, pairing activities. Countertransference within such a group would, by the same token, denote a leader's acting out *with* the group, i.e., a deviation from his "asymmetric" abstinent role. Typically, such "countertransference" could occur in three major ways: first, the group therapist lets himself be forced into the role of the all-giving and all-knowing father-mother, i.e., he tries to satisfy the group's excessive and regressive dependency needs; second, he confirms through his actual behavior the group's perception of him as a controlling, authoritarian intruder who must be fought or be fled; or, third, he allows or covertly encourages excessive pairing relations within the group. All three countertransference patterns lead to characteristic impasses in group therapy, as group therapists well know—unless they are quickly recognized and checked.

"TRANSFERENCE" AND "COUNTERTRANSFERENCE" IN FAMILY GROUPS

Families are groups and as such appear not exempt from the above considerations and principles. However, as groups they are also so unique that they almost require a totally new script. And this applies, above all, to the meanings of transference and countertransference in family therapy.

Two features of families are here crucial:

First, families are the opposites of transient, "ad hoc" groups who lack a common history and a mutual involvement beyond that which their group relationship generates. Rather, families share such history, and their members have been and will be, fatefully and enduringly, enmeshed with each other.

Second, families do not primarily reveal transferences and countertransferences as found in either dyadic relations or groups. For transactional phenomena in families, whatever their specific content and source, reflect, foremostly, one fact—*that transferences originate within families. It is family transactions which give rise to those relational patterns which* *later, inappropriately and repetitively, are transferred to non-family contexts.**

These two central family facts—that family members are fatefully enmeshed with each other, and that transferences originate within their sphere—account for the importance of one phenomenon that is central to the theory and practice of family therapy and for our conceptualization of transference and countertransference processes in families: the existence of family myths.

Family myths, as here intended, have been extensively described and illustrated by Ferreira (1963), who emphasized their homeostatic function. He maintained that "the family myth is to the relationship what the defense is to the individual." I myself have recently outlined the varying functions and structures of family myths (Stierlin, 1973).

Here it must suffice to say that family myths fulfill the major function of providing a shared formulation which makes some sense out of the family members' involvement with, and their rights and obligations vis-à-vis, each other. Thus, myths serve cognitive needs (they give a—more or less—coherent picture of "where the family is at"), relational needs (they anchor the members in mutual relatedness), as well as needs for interpersonal justice (they assign blame or grant exculpation to certain members) . In brief, they provide cognitive, relational and ethical meaning and are therefore affectively charged. To make this clearer, let us look at one particular family myth which centered around the "badness" of an alcoholic father (who happened to be no longer in the picture).

This father, so the myth went, had malevolently deserted his faithful wife and loving children. Therefore, all members agreed that he needed to be shunned and castigated, and they all shared in the belief that this bad, deserting, alcoholic father was innately corrupt, irresponsible, in brief, the scum of the earth. This father's "desertion" occurred approximately ten years before the family entered therapy. Meanwhile, the mother had remarried. Her new husband, the children's stepfather, had

---

* Closer inspection reveals that transferences originate in different, though related, families. For example, the presenting parents had their formative, transference-generating relationships as children to their parents, whereas their children, whose relational patterns they (the parents) fatefully shaped (and still shape), will in turn have an impact on their own children, etc. Given such a multigenerational perspective, so-called "parentifications" can be viewed as transferences within families or as *trans-generational transferences*: parents "transfer" to their children those expectations, unfulfilled longings, needs for nutriment, wishes for revenge, etc., which derived from their own child-parent interactions.

also come to believe that the family's current difficulties—such as the mother's depression, the oldest girl's promiscuity, the boy's school difficulties, etc.—were essentially due to this father's desertion. Thus, this myth tried to make sense of this family's basic nature, relatedness, history, and plight, as it assigned blame to one member (the father) while exculpating all others.

Gradually, though, this myth was punctured as it became known that the father's "desertion" was in part engineered by the mother, who then had a love affair with her boss. More and more this father came to be seen not so much as an irresponsible runaway, but as a pathetic evictee who again and again clamored to re-enter the family, yet each time was rebuffed. As a result of the exploratory family therapy, a more complex view of the family's history emerged, and each member's merits and demerits appeared more evenly balanced.

When we focus on specific transference-countertransference dynamics in families, we find, thus, that myths have characteristic effects on them. First, they distort as well as disguise these dynamics—to the family members, as well as to outsiders. In the above case, for example, the myth almost totally ignored or obfuscated the nature of those most formative, primary relationships in this family which later gave rise to compulsive, repetitive transference patterns in individual members. For while the myth directed everybody's attention to the father's desertion, it left unrecognized and unexplored the mother's intrusive and controlling relationship with her daughter (which later became a central focus in the family therapy). At the same time, the myth painted a distorted picture of the members' involvement with each other: while it scapegoated the absent father, it white-washed all other members.

Second, to the extent that this myth could be "sold" to outsiders, including family therapists, it invited from them a typical "countertransference" response—one that condemned the father and exculpated the other family members. Had such "countertransference" response actually occurred, it would not have been a reaction to the family's transference (be this from individual members or the family as a whole), but rather an unwitting reaction to, as well as acceptance of, the family's collaborative and distortive script of the family drama. As such, it would have proven a stumbling block to family therapy, attributable chiefly to a "blind spot"—i.e., a lack of perceptiveness and objectivity—in the family therapist.

Transferences in families, to sum this up, are not quick to develop. As relational patterns, they appear locked up within the family system and pressed into the distortive strait jacket of myths, which prevent them from being pried loose and experienced and recognized as transferences. This contrasts with the easily mobilized transferences found in many neurotic patients, described by Ferenczi (1909) and many others, and in the earlier-mentioned ad hoc groups. Consequently, also, the term countertransference must take on a new meaning in family therapy.

COUNTERTRANSFERENCE AS A DEVIATION FROM "INVOLVED IMPARTIALITY"

To grasp this new meaning, we must keep in mind that for the family therapist the primary issue is not so much one of reacting inappropriately to the family members' transference, *but rather of dealing with their defenses—particularly myths—which hide and distort, to the family members and to the therapist, these members' deeper, formative, and trans-ference-generating relations.*

This implies that the family therapist must move into the family system, but not with a hammer, as it were. Rather, he should do this in ways which are consonant with an increasing build-up of trust with *all* family members; he must involve himself meaningfully and empathically with each one of them; yet in so doing he must remain fair to all. This does not mean he must be obsessed with whether he gives each member exactly the same amount of attention, but that he, in the long run, makes each member feel understood and appreciated.

I. Boszormenyi-Nagy (1972) spoke of the family therapist's multi-directional partiality—a partiality afforded individual members, yet one that goes out in all directions. I would like to speak of the therapist's *involved impartiality,* thereby emphasizing the therapist's basic fairness, as maintained under conditions of increasing involvement with each member. While he tries to gain each member's trust, the therapist explores and thereby punctures the family myths. This allows him and the members to reassess basic family dynamics and to evaluate ever more fairly each member's rights, obligations, and accountability. In this process, the family therapist must be active, as Wynne (1965), Boszormenyi-Nagy and Spark (1973), and others have pointed out; but his activity is less a matter of his style (silent therapists can sometimes be more effectively active than many talkative ones) than of his concern and dynamic involvement. Yet, while active, he must always let himself be guided by what the family presents as its problem, that is, he must not be ahead of the family, and must not let his interventions or interpretations be dictated by what *he* thinks the family's problem is.

To the extent that trust develops, transferences are pried loose from within the family and the therapist will become their most likely recipient. Once this happens, classical views and formulations as to the development of transference-countertransference reactions become more applicable. We observe how parents increasingly relate to the therapist as they related to their own parents, while their children bring to bear on him those relational patterns which originated in *their* parent relationships. As he turns increasingly into a target for individual transferences, the therapist tries to provide each member with a corrective emotional experience, even though he might often not be able to deal exhaustively with the transference reactions he elicits. At the same time, it becomes often more difficult, but also more important, that he maintain his overall attitude of "involved impartiality."

Boszormenyi-Nagy (1972) has described how the therapist is often "parentified" by parents who, until then, tended to parentify their children. By letting himself become parentified in their stead—i.e., by offering himself as an object for those longings, repair needs, retaliatory impulses, etc., which originated vis-à-vis the parents' own parents but until now had been displaced onto their adolescent children—the therapist often has a striking immediate "liberative" impact on the latter: they stop being troublesome problem adolescents, get more easily and constructively involved with peers, and in the family sessions become more helpful, thoughtful, and communicative.

Thus, I define countertransference in families operationally as any deviation from a therapeutic position of involved impartiality, as outlined above.

PHASES IN THE DEVELOPMENT OF FAMILY TRANSFERENCE AND COUNTERTRANSFERENCE

Such deviation reflects always the phase of the therapeutic process, and derives its specific meaning chiefly from what transpires in *two phases*: a first phase during which the therapist, by building and using trust, penetrates the distortive strait jacket of family myths, thereby shaking up the family homeostasis and prying loose the members'—mainly parent-derived and parentifying—transferences; and a second phase during which he increasingly becomes a target for such "unhooked" transferences, to which he then reacts.

These two phases represent ideal types rather than lawfully unfolding phenomena. Certain families—mainly those which are amorphous and fragmented—appear highly transference-prone from the beginning, whereas other families seem so tightly locked up within themselves that they resist to the very end any meaningful "unhooking" of individual transferences. Ordinarily, though, the two phases can be clearly observed.

During each phase, the therapist's "countertransference" might be a response to taxing treatment challenges and then serve primarily as a source of information about the family or some member, or it might primarily reflect certain defenses, personality traits, growth lacunae, or "blind spots" in himself which interfere with his therapeutic task—i.e., become stumbling blocks—and then require corrective action.

"Overactive" or "passive" therapists, for example, may reveal different "countertransference" problems during the two phases. Thus, an overactive therapist during the first phase might become a manipulative interventionist who "shakes up" the family, but fails to build trust, whereas the more passive—frequently psychoanalytically trained—therapist may miss his chance to move dynamically into the family.

During the second phase, the overactive and passive therapists may fail in different ways to serve as receptive targets for unhooked individual transference reactions—the overactive therapist by dispensing cheap consolation or advice, the passive therapist by remaining detached and remote.

SPECIFIC "COUNTERTRANSFERENCE" PROBLEMS IN THE TREATMENT
OF FAMILIES WITH ADOLESCENTS

Adolescents, with their specific strengths, weaknesses, and problems, introduce a further complexity into an already complex treatment situation. Most important from the vantage point here adopted is the centripetal momentum of adolescence—the tendency of adolescents to move out of the family field and to thereby upset the family homeostasis. This implies, among other things, multileveled conflicts of missions and loyalties which I have described elsewhere (1972, and, with Ravenscroft, 1972). It is, above all, conflicts of loyalties which tend to elicit characteristic "countertransference" responses from family therapists—that is, tempt them to deviate from a position of "involved impartiality." Instead of maintaining such a position, they side with one party against the other, for example, with parent against child, child against parent, or one generation against the other, thereby deepening the members' loyalty conflicts and problems.

Let us, then, consider more closely how such countertransference, revealed in a taking of sides by the therapist, might show up in the family therapy with adolescents.

The Therapist Siding with the "Sick" Victimized Adolescent

Such siding seems often irresistible, when a perceptive family therapist realizes how certain parents "dump" their own "sickness" and disturbance on their adolescent offspring via projective identification. In so doing, these parents define the latter to himself as sick, depressed, anxious, etc., whereas they consider themselves as healthy and reasonable. This process I have elsewhere defined as delegating in the service of the parents' self-observation and conscience (with Ravenscroft, 1972). When such a family comes to see a psychiatrist, a showdown situation has usually developed. At this juncture in the family's life, an adolescent offspring is expected to deliver the living proof of being *the* sick family member by acquiescing to patient status or even to hospitalization. Particularly, certain mothers of schizophrenic patients, as described by L. Hill (1955), T. Lidz et al. (1965), and others, have gained a reputation as devastating victimizers of their adolescent children. Hence the concept, highly charged and problematical, of the "schizophrenogenic mother" who disowns onto her captive child her own anxiety, depression, confusion, or badness.

Instead of—overtly or covertly—taking sides with the victim against his parental victimizer—this constituting a countertransference reaction, according to the above operational definition—the therapist must now maintain his involved impartiality in ways which also do justice to the victimizing parent. To do so, he needs to realize the immense power the willing "victim" frequently wields over his parent. Boszormenyi-Nagy (1972, and, with Spark, 1973) has well described this process. He pointed out that this willing victim is in a strategic position to operate the guilt lever over his parents by delivering himself to them as the living proof of their failure or badness as parents. The therapist who consciously or unconsciously sides with this victim against his parents stirs their guilt ever more deeply, for he now supports with his medical authority the patient's masochistic power ploy. A parent can usually discharge this increased guilt only by assuming an even harsher punitive and blaming —that is, victimizing—stance vis-à-vis the adolescent who, his own unconscious guilt rising, will be driven to further live up to his parents' victimization of him, thereby deadlocking him and them ever more tightly in a "spiral of negative mutuality" (Stierlin, 1969, and, with Levi and Savard, 1971).

Such "siding" with the adolescent victim may derive from an unrecognized and unworked-through separation problem of the therapist. Unwittingly, he might need to make the patient's parents feel bad for things which his (the therapist's) own parents did to him. Also, he might—again unconsciously—revel in the role of rescuer of mistreated victims, and in this role discharge righteous, though displaced, indignation against the victim's oppressors. Such combination of rescue drive and "righteous indignation" may for a while "vitalize" his overall therapeutic work, but will inevitably bring about its ruin.

The Therapist Siding with the "Rebellious" Adolescent

Overtly, this rebellious adolescent—i.e., one who curses his parents with four-letter words, does not follow orders, stays out late in the night, dresses and acts like a bum, etc.—may seem to wage a battle for independence in which he asks his therapist's support. Covertly, though, he usually hangs onto immature forms of dependence and conforms to his parents' (conflictual and ambiguous) expectations. Not infrequently he enacts—again via projective identification—his parent's disowned rebellious impulses as their loyal delegate (see Johnson and Szurek, 1952; Stierlin, 1972). Whatever the major motivational dynamics, the therapist is usually ill-advised to serve as a spokesman for his "rebellion." This becomes ever more evident when such "rebellion" is acted out via sexual promiscuity, dangerous motorcycling, or drug use. A therapist, in secret alliance with an adolescent "rebel," may empathically share the latter's exposure to contradictory messages and loss of needed identity support structures, but usually is unable to help him—unless he dissolves the alliance and returns to an involved impartiality.

The motivational dynamics in the therapist can vary here; yet usually they point to his own unresolved problems of adolescent individuation and separation. In particular, this seems to hold true for certain young therapists who appear still close to, if not stuck in, their own late adolescence. Through their dress, e.g., slightly frayed jeans, and manner of hippie talk, they document visibly their identification with the protesting younger generation. Having not yet achieved a more mature dependence (or independence, if you wish) in relation to their own parents, they recruit their patients to unwittingly and vicariously continue their own "rebellious" struggle.

The Therapist Siding with the Victimized Parent

Such siding with the victimized parent differs from the empathic appreciation of the plight of the victimized victimizer, described above, and represents a "countertransference pattern." The siding therapist over-identifies—again without being aware he does it—with the "poor, well-meaning, decent" parent whom the "spoiled, obstreperous" adolescent has pushed into a corner. He unwittingly shares sentiments, articulated and exploited by the Ronald Reagans and Spiro Agnews, of toughness and "law and order" in dealing with the "Spock-marked" generation. In siding with the victimized parent, he may encourage the latter to drastically punish or reject the adolescent, rationalizing such a stance as "firmness" or "setting of limits." But rather than helping the parents to stand firm, he only supports the rejecting, hostile side in their ambivalence, thereby courting disaster; for the more the parents reject and punish, the more they also alienate their adolescent. Consuming themselves with guilt, the parents often waver and shift from over-strictness to over-permissiveness. At the same time, they make themselves more vulnerable to their adolescent victim's masochistic power ploys, as earlier described. And again the result is a "negative mutuality" which blocks the process of individuation-separation for parents and adolescent offspring.

Therapists who unwittingly side with parents tend in my experience to be older than therapists who side with adolescents. Often they have children in the adolescent age range with whom they unsuccessfully struggle. At closer inspection, they, too, appear burdened with problems that often date back to their own adolescence. As a rule, this adolescence seems to have been difficult and deprived. We may discover that their own parents treated them then in the same manner in which they, as parents, now treat *their* adolescent children. They cannot help taking their children—as well as their adolescent patients—to task for what *their* parents once did to them.

Unwitting Competitive Displacement of Parents

Here the therapist installs himself unwittingly as a more effective parent than the adolescent's actual parents. Typically, he is unaware of how this affects the displaced parent. A recent study of our group at the Family Studies Section of the Adult Psychiatry Branch, National Institute of Mental Health, illuminated this problem (see Levi, Stierlin, Savard, 1972). In follow-up interviews, conducted on previously treated families, we found that a number of fathers, during and subsequent to family therapy, appeared to have become more depressed and less effective parents. These fathers, we came to realize, had for some time been suffering from chronic, insidious depression, deriving largely from their unresolved mid-life crises. Wrapped up in their depression, they had subjected themselves to incessant harsh and negative self-assessment which found them wanting as fathers, professionals, and providers. When this happened, they withdrew emotionally from their adolescent sons. Instead of engaging them in a "loving fight," urgently needed for the delineation of their (the sons') budding male identities, they left them stranded in a relational vacuum. From this vacuum the sons would then turn to their mother's emotional orbit, frequently becoming spoiled and infantilized in the process. Lacking the counteracting force of a father, *against* whom they could bump and *with* whom they could identify, their oedipal problems intensified.

These fathers, their self-esteem shaken, could not help comparing themselves unfavorably to their younger, more energetic, and more effective male therapists. Rather than identifying with these therapists and learning their parenting skills and effectiveness, they experienced further proof of their own failure and unworthiness.

In reappraising this outcome, we realized that the therapists had here also deviated from a position of "involved impartiality" and thus had engaged in characteristic "countertransference." This time, however, it was less a matter of taking sides with some family member (or members) against another member, than of not sufficiently and tactfully appreciating the side of one member—i.e., that of the father. In brief, the therapists were insufficiently tuned to the emotional dynamics and plights of these middle-aged fathers.*

Closer inspection points also here to recurrent, unresolved "adolescent" problems of therapists. These therapists tend to displace parents, while unwittingly they reenact an earlier competitive and/or oedipal struggle. Typically, they need to take charge in a sometimes unreflective and even controlling way. While activity of family therapists is crucial, as indicated earlier, such "taking charge" is often detrimental to the parent and the progress of therapy, because it amounts to an humiliating oedipal dethronement of a parent by a younger, more successful rival.

---

* This raises the question of how well any family therapist not yet middle-aged can empathize with such middle-aged parents. Martin Buber, during his last stay in Washington, is said to have stated: "No one under the age of 45 should be a therapist" (Weigert, 1973). This might be even more true for family therapists.

The family background of one young family therapist seemed here illuminating. The oldest of several children and his mother's favorite son, he had from an early age taken over much of his father's role in controlling the younger children and supervising the large household. Professionally he had become more successful than his father, who had held lowly positions throughout his life. Thus, this very gifted and hard-driving therapist won a striking oedipal triumph over his father. However, this triumph remained shallow in at least some respects. As a family therapist, he could not help—albeit compulsively and unwittingly—competing with, and winning out over, any new father who came into sight. This "countertransference" problem, which also affected his non-therapeutic relationships, made a later personal analysis advisable.

Analogous to the above is the compulsive need of certain female therapists to be a more effective—i.e., more nurturant, giving and loving—mother than is the adolescent's actual mother. Competition with this mother may here also reinforce the wish to rescue the victimized adolescent—an endeavor most likely to fail for the reasons already given.

SOME CONCLUSIONS

I have tried to show that the therapist's countertransference in families takes on a meaning different from what we find in individual analysis and group therapy. Above everything, the family therapist must be able to practice an "involved impartiality," and countertransference in families can operationally be defined as a deviation from such therapeutic position. When we look more closely at the dynamics of such deviation, we often find, as we do in other countertransference contexts, that information-providing and stumbling block aspects interweave. Where the latter dominate, we are alerted to "growth lacunae" and "blind spots" in the therapist. These growth lacunae and blind spots often reflect difficulties the therapist had, or still has, in growing up and in separating from his own family, and frequently date back to his own adolescence.

Freud recommended the didactic (or training) analysis of the psychoanalyst as the best—and perhaps only—method to eliminate his blind spots. From the vantage point adopted in this chapter, a similar didactic (and therapeutic) family therapy would be indicated for the therapist of families. Such "training family therapy" is now, at least in some quarters, being recommended for the younger generation of family therapists while other family therapists still consider it impractical or outright impossible. I believe an individual therapeutic or training analysis can substitute for such desirable family therapy—at least to some extent. (After all, an individual psychoanalysis brings us into touch with our formative family relations—albeit now shaped by the nature and vicissitudes of the psychoanalytic transference.) Apart from such individual analysis for the family therapist, the co-therapy with, and observation by, colleagues can help us to increase our awareness of our growth lacunae, blind spots, and resulting countertransference reactions. And there is, finally, our experience with our own families—our family of origin as well as our family of procreation—which may provide us with vital insights and opportunities for growth that eventually serve to counteract, if not eliminate, undesirable countertransference processes.

REFERENCES

ARGELANDER, H. (1972). Gruppenprozesse/Wege zur Anwendung der Psychoanalyse. In *Behandlung, Lehre und Forschung*. Reinbeck: Rowohlt.

BION, W. (1961). *Experiences in Groups*. London: Tavistock.

BOSZORMENYI-NAGY, I. (1972). Loyalty implications of the transference model in psychotherapy. *Archives of General Psychiatry*, 27:374-380.

BOSZORMENYI-NAGY, I., and SPARK, G. (1973). *Invisible Loyalties*. New York: Hoeber & Harper.

COHEN, M. B. (1952). Countertransference and anxiety. *Psychiatry*, 15:231-243.

EZRIEL, H. (1950). A psycho-analytic approach to group treatment. *British Journal of Medical Psychology*, 23:59-74.

FERENCZI, S. (1916). Introjection and transference (1909). *Sex in Psychoanalysis*. Boston: Gorham Press.

FERREIRA, A. (1963). Family myths and homeostasis. *Archives of General Psychiatry*, 9:457-463.

FREUD, S. (1957). The future prospects of psycho-analytic therapy (1910). *Standard Edition*, 11:139-151. London: Hogarth Press.

FREUD, S. (1955). Studies on Hysteria (1895). *Standard Edition*, 2:48-305. London: Hogarth Press.

FREUD, S. (1953). Fragment of an analysis of a case of hysteria (1905). *Standard Edition*, 7:3-122. London: Hogarth Press.

FREUD, S. (1955). Group psychology and the analysis of the ego (1921). *Standard Edition*, 18:67-143. London: Hogarth Press.

FROMM-REICHMANN, F. (1950). *Principles of Intensive Psychotherapy*. Chicago: University of Chicago Press.

GROTJAHN, M. (1953). Special aspects of countertransference in analytic group psychotherapy. *International Journal of Group Psychotherapy*, 3:407-416.

HILL, L. (1955). *Psychotherapeutic Intervention in Schizophrenia*. Chicago: University of Chicago Press.

JOHNSON, A., and SZUREK, S. A. (1952). The genesis of antisocial acting out in children and adults. *Psychoanalytic Quarterly*, 21:323-343.

LEVI, L. D., STIERLIN, H., and SAVARD, R. J. (1972). Fathers and sons: The interlocking crises of integrity and identity. *Psychiatry*, 35:48-56.

LIDZ, T., CORNELISON, A. R., SINGER, M. T., SCHAFER, S., and FLECK, S. (1965). The mothers of schizophrenic patients. In *Schizophrenia and the Family*, T. Lidz, S. Fleck, and A. R. Cornelison, eds. New York: International Universities Press.

tional modalities, such as group or individual therapy for the adolescent; or may remain the primary or sole form of therapeutic intervention with an adolescent and his family by regular weekly family interviews over a period of many months.

There is no doubt that a disturbed adolescent needs much assistance in breaking his ambivalent family ties as he strives for identity and independence. Some therapists feel this can only be done by his developing a highly confidential one-to-one relationship with an adult outside the family, his psychotherapist. Some psychotherapists are unique in their capacity to rise above ensuing familial resistances to the establishment of such out-of-the-family relationships. They are able to develop with the teenager a most powerful new corrective relationship. However, I believe that in most situations the familial resistances will prevail, block, and overcome progress. As a child enters adolescence, these parental resistances to his forward development can be quite severe. For instance, at no time in a woman's life is her own identity more threatened than at that point when her maternal role must give way in light of her last child's adolescent maturity. This is particularly so if her marriage is not a rewarding one. Mothers at such points of personal crisis may unwittingly hold on to their teenage sons and daughters, stifling their psychosocial growth. Seeing the adolescent together with his parents allows for a mutual working through of these resistances. Some of the questions raised by those who are reluctant to see the adolescent with his family include: Will family therapy help individuation or promote an even greater continued symbiosis? Will not such family meetings result in a break of confidentiality with the adolescent? The complex familial field that surrounds an adolescent often perplexes the clinician. This perplexity overwhelms many therapists to the point of avoiding working with adolescents and of adopting a stance of therapeutic nihilism. Some teachers avoid the perplexities by presenting students with an oversimplified exposure to adolescent psychiatry, primarily a one-to-one dyadic approach. Varying flexible and multitreatment techniques are not sufficiently introduced early enough in the student's or resident's training. Unfortunately, the reassurance that a beginning student attains from working in the one-to-one, easy to control, uncovering psychotherapeutic approach with adults often collapses when he faces an adolescent and the multiforces within the family that he, the therapist, cannot control. I should like to suggest that therapists who feel in control while working exclusively in the dyadic one-to-one relationship with an adolescent actually have very little control, merely the illusion of it. Whittling away goes on behind the scenes in the form of overt and subtle sabotage within the family field.

I should like to discuss the indications for family therapy in adolescent psychiatry, both for assessment and for treatment. Attention will be paid to the most serious dilemma for the adolescent and his family, the age-old conflict between autonomy and individuation as it comes into conflict with dependency-control attachments, particularly in the next to impossible to treat symbiotic type family. The author encourages flexibility of approach within the total treatment program for the adolescent, a flexibility that includes therapeutically timed mixtures of one-to-one therapy and family treatment.

MAJOR CONFLICTS OF ADOLESCENCE

Before attending to indications and contraindications for family interviewing techniques, I should like to briefly review some of those major conflicts of adolescence for which families can either offer resolution or stifling perpetuation.

Independence Versus Dependency Attachments

The adolescent, in his struggle to achieve freedom from his family, often threatens, within himself and his parents, very primitive fears of object loss and separation from symbiotic involvements. Brown (1969) indicated how the transactional field of the family is often used to reaffirm and preserve the internal infantile object constellation in an effort to ward off fantasied separation grief and anxiety. Minuchin (1971) described how in working with very close-knit families the therapist must be aware of the powerful familial forces that impede maturity for the adolescent. He further stressed the need for clinicians to find effective ways of overcoming these forces.

Today, many adolescents attempt to solve their own intrapsychic and their family's problems over independence and dependency attachments by leaving home at an early age. Unfortunately, what often results from such attempts to jar loose from the family is a state of pseudomaturation. The underlying sense of weakness and object loss frequently persists and represents itself in a growing need for drugs and new attachments within hippie-type crash pads or communes (Williams, 1970). Such dependency attachments to peers—without the development of significant mutuality and intimacy—can result in a group of adolescents holding together like orphans in a storm, merely playing at the game of maturity.

Some succeed in developing, in spite of the game; others fail and remain symbolically attached to their families, through the fantasied family objects in their new surrogate peer parents. Williams (1970) described how adolescents in a hippie commune display an exquisite attempt to work through the attachment-autonomy conflict with the use of drugs. He offers examples in which the adolescent parent nurses his peer child back to health from a bad trip. At a later point, that same former child-patient becomes the mother and nurses his former peer parent back to health from a similar bad trip. Unfortunately, very little in the way of sustained day-to-day experiences in maintaining a role of growing leadership seems to occur.

Recrudescence of Oedipal Conflicts

The sexual conflicts stirred up within the adolescent, by nature of his physical and psychosexual growth, often lead to the development of dramatic distancing mechanisms between parents and their sons and daughters. Mutual fears of fantasied hetero- and homosexual erotization of the parent-child relationships are often represented in extreme defensive hostile pushing-away maneuvers in some families. In others, the parents become overtly involved in the sexuality of their sons and daughters. This may be reflected in either direct seductive contact, or in subtle cueing mechanisms, wherein a mother, for example, using the rationalization of instilling "a healthy wholesome attitude," overeducates her daughter about sex and elicits detailed descriptions from her young adolescent daughter of sexual fantasies and encounters.

The role of the parents and siblings in the reappearance of threatening incestuous fantasies in adolescence has received little emphasis in the literature. Family interviewing techniques offer opportunities to observe directly those subtle seductive stimuli from sisters and brothers, as well as from parents, usually not gleaned from sessions with the parents alone. The adolescent faced with symbolic or real incestuous provocation often finds it difficult to sublimate his feelings in the direction of nonsexual familial intimacy experiences. This is, in most families today, owing to a lack of experiences with intimate sharing of feelings between parent and child, after the initial maternal-infant symbiosis and parental-preschooler closeness. The adolescent is therefore trapped. He either leaves and looks for intimacy outside his home, or he remains within the family and suffers the fantasied and/or part reality threat of massive regression to those types of early oral and anal intimacy experiences he knew as a young child and as an infant. Should he choose to leave home, in an effort to seek love and intimacy, he has very little intimacy capacity with which to sustain himself. He often winds up substituting pseudo-sexual intimacies and the pseudointimacy of the hippie or drug scene.

Integration of Angry Affect

In adolescence, significant real physical strength is available for the first time. Too, the capacity for calculation related to carrying out of crimes and physical harm is readily available. Adolescents are often frightened by their rage and destructive potential, particularly in relation to their parents. The rage often relates to inner struggles over autonomy and is projected onto the parents. Should the parents have intense problems regarding letting go, the projection, of course, becomes much easier to accomplish and more readily fixated. At other times, the teenager's rage represents a defense against emerging positive erotic feelings toward parents or siblings. Completely separating the adolescent's therapy from his family's therapy may parallel the negative effect of a teenager's premature leaving of home, as far as rage is concerned. When the adolescent leaves home (made easy today by the availability of hippie communes or crashpads, which will provide food and shelter), he does not have an opportunity to fight out certain rage-inducing conflicts with his parents and siblings. Fighting it out can help the adolescent test the extent and limitations of his own murderous rage in terms of potential action, as well as the extent and limitations of his parents' and siblings' murderous rage in terms of potential danger. Some adolescent peer groups maintain an ideology of love. The proclamation, "We love everyone, including the parents who hassle us!" may serve as a defense against the eruption of repressed or suppressed feelings of rage toward family members. Family therapy offers a safe and constructive setting in which to fight it out.

Much can be inferred regarding that portion of an adolescent's problem with angry affect, which stems from familial relationships, by seeing parents in separate diagnostic or therapeutic sessions. Family interviews, however, which include the parents and adolescent together, offer an *in vivo* opportunity to determine whether the rage relates to defensive paranoid projection on the part of the adolescent, or to reality-oriented parental precipitants. Such a differential assessment helps in determining intrapsychic fixation and potential for the later handling of rage feelings once separation from the family does occur. Brown (1964) described an example of parental stimulation of inappropriate anger in a young teenage boy with self-destructive tendencies. In several interviews, which included the boy, his mother, father, and sister, a fascinating interplay between the boy's problem with inner controls and familial interpersonal relations was elicited. In part the therapist was able to observe how the father's avoidance of decisive discipline helped to perpetuate the youngster's problem with controls. He was also able to observe, within the nuances of the familial interactions, how the father and son made a regressive alliance, a focal symbiosis, in which they both retreated from their phallically feared mother and in which the father used his son both as a retreat and as a symbiolic expression of his own rage toward his wife.

Identity and Capacity for Intimacy

The adolescent's capacity for intimacy and his ego identity—his separateness—are affected by his family's attitude toward his individuation. Some families with very powerful familial identities display a wholesome working togetherness, but unwittingly squelch the individual identities of the various family members. Adolescents sometimes flee from such families in a desperate attempt to achieve a sense of individuality. Once with a new family peer group, they are supersensitive and on guard in relation to fears of their becoming possessed and of losing separateness. A question pertinent to the field of family therapy is, "Can an adolescent work through his struggle between his desire for intimacy and his fear of loss of individuation, within the context of family therapy sessions, or separate from his family in an individual new intimate one-to-one relationship with a therapist?" My own bias is in the direction of a flexible combination of both modalities for adolescent therapy. The family can often be helped to encourage the teenager toward independent individuation; the teenager's role in undermining that potential encouragement from his parents is most observable and available for confrontation in family meetings.

INDICATIONS FOR FAMILY THERAPY WITH ADOLESCENTS

Assessment

Regardless of the treatment modality eventually decided on for an adolescent, family interviews during the diagnostic phase help the therapist to understand the multitude of outer forces perpetuating and contributing to the adolescent's internal conflicts. Family interviews can be helpful during the initial workup, as well as at major points of resistance, during an ongoing individual treatment. One or two initial diagnostic family interviews help the therapist with prognostic considerations. He is able to determine more accurately those factors in the family that will serve as major resistances to the uncovering work of one-to-one individual therapy with the adolescent. There are at times certain affects hidden within the adolescent, related to past tragic family traumas. These affects may be continually held down via subtle parental cues, in an effort to protect the parent from the pain of affective recall, memory, or expression. For example, a severely depressed 13-year-old boy was desperately in need of psychotherapy to help relieve him of self-destructive tendencies and his gloomy preoccupation with the hopelessness of failing peer relationships. Seeing the boy and mother in separate diagnostic sessions elicited historical material about the father's death several years earlier. Neither mother nor son showed the slightest affect while presenting the material about the father's sudden death. Mother's monotone presentation was noteworthy. When seeing the boy and mother together in a family interview, it was striking to note that whenever the boy attempted to discuss his feelings about his father's death, he immediately evoked from his mother a gentle but definitive prohibition against further ventilation. The boy's eyes would well up with tears as he would start to say with sadness that he "remembered when his father . . . "; the mother would immediately say something to the effect of, "Your father was a good man and it isn't proper to talk about him." Even when it was apparent that the boy was about to say something positive about his father, the mother would again prohibit such expression by changing the subject or by indicating the potential hurt she would feel if one "dredged up the past." In this particular case, a series of family interviews was helpful in freeing the mother to give her son permission to uncover and ventilate his feelings of depression and rage about the loss of his father. One might have attempted to get this boy to reach the same point in individual therapy. I feel, however, that in so doing one could readily create new conflicts for the youngster, as he would have to blindly struggle with his conflict over loyalty to his own wish for relief and his mother's wish for continued burial of affects. Paul and Grosser (1965) described the values of uncovering such buried affects from the traumatic past during family interviews.

Diagnostic family interviews help to assess whether the intrapsychic distortions of the adolescent are firmly fixated and resistant to changes within the environment, or whether such distortions are still in a state of fluidity and primarily reinforced, daily, by parental cueing. I recently treated a 16-year-old girl with severe anorexia nervosa. The original diagnostic workup reflected some of the classical conflicts over fear of separation from mother and fear of her adult female sexual impulses. In individual diagnostic sessions, Marie tearfully told of how her wish to have a boyfriend, and how her dreams of sex with boys made her feel "trampy." She was openly anxious as she discussed her desire to eventually live away from home. In the parents' separate diagnostic history-taking interview, the mother convincingly indicated her own healthy approach toward sex, as far as her daughter was concerned, and stressed how she encouraged Marie to date and to learn about sex from both books and from questions put to the parents. In marked contrast to the tone of the individual sessions was one family interview, in which the question of Marie's dating and leaving home came up. As Marie's tears and anxiety level lessened, she began to talk of a boy she met at school who wanted to take her out. Marie's father blanched; her mother sat forward and said, "What do you know about him?" She then turned to me and said, "Doctor, we know that there are some nice boys, but my father was a policeman, you know, and I've learned about all the rapes and murders that go on, particularly with young girls; you never know what a boy is really like; he may just be putting on a friendly front!" The next day in an individual session with me, Marie appeared extremely frightened. She described how she had not eaten all day and how uncertain she felt about her feelings in relationship to boys and dating. This is a striking example of an observable direct influence by the parents on the unresolved autonomy and sexual conflicts of an adolescent.

When doing family interviewing, one has an opportunity to note such overt as well as certain subtle cueing mechanisms. At times mothers and fathers will discuss with seeming frankness their concerns about hetero- and homosexuality and will, at times, show zealous interest in their adolescent son's or daughter's sexual activities. The family therapist is in a position to see those cues that admonish or prematurely encourage sexual involvement. These cues are often missed in the more traditional diagnostic interview.

One has an excellent opportunity in family meetings to observe directly double-bind communications. For example, a 15-year-old boy lived alone with his divorced mother. In her initial individual intake session, the mother complained of her son's lack of friends; she wanted the clinic to "help him get out of his shell and make more meaningful friendships." In a diagnostic family meeting, the boy discussed his wish for friends, but added his concerns about his mother's loneliness. Mother broke into tears, saying, "I want you to go out, you need to be away from me, somehow I will survive; it is important for you to have your own life!" The boy was torn in that his mother had given him permission, but at the same time had indirectly indicated that she might die without him.

Family interviews during the diagnostic phase often elicit marital disharmony or potential disharmony, which is covered up by the scapegoating of the problem teenager. Frequently, one of the siblings is the first to uncover the disharmony. Brown (1970), in his description of family therapy, indicated how family meetings can promote a readiness to deal with change in the marital relationship. He particularly noted how siblings who are not directly caught up in the pathologic family dyads may move this process along. The scapegoated problem adolescent serves to ward off a threatened potential break in the family equilibrium should the parents' underlying hatred or intimacy deficit be brought to the surface. The designated teenage patient often loyally accepts his role as the sick one, though ashamed of it, in an effort to hold his parents and family together. In family meetings, one can observe the exquisite and precise timing of some of the shifting of attention to the teenager's problems, as the therapist or one of the family gets close to touching on the underlying marital conflict. A sibling may point out the lack of time mother and father spend together, or the lack of romantic feelings between the parents. Suddenly, and apparently out of context, the designated patient or one of the parents will draw attention to the adolescent's symptoms. In several family treatment situations, we have noted how symptom complexes such as aggressive behavior disorders, predelinquency, and poor school performance abate once the parents are able to ventilate their anxieties about the instability of their marriage. In these cases, the treatment of choice is often conjoint marital therapy without any therapy necessary for the adolescent.

In diagnostic family interviews one obtains a sense of whether a family will be of help in attempts to reverse an adolescent's intrapsychic distortions. In an interview with a 16-year-old boy with sleep problems, school failures, and a lack of friends, the youngster indicated severe conflicts regarding his wish to go to a nonparochial school. He feared his father, a long-time religious devotee, would condemn his wish to attend a coed school. He further feared that he would bear the brunt of peer ridicule if he wore his religious skullcap in a coed setting. The father, in a meeting with the boy and the therapist, shared his own mixed feelings about the matter, but convincingly encouraged the boy to go to a coed school and to remove his skullcap. It became clear that much of the work to be done in individual therapy would need to focus on the boy's underlying fears of sexuality, and that his father would probably be an ally, or at least not a sabotaging agent.

Overcoming Resistances

In individual or group therapy, the clinician often faces what appears to be a major resistance to continue treatment. Those of us who work a great deal with adolescents are all too familiar with the frequency of missed sessions, latenesses, and the boredom that often sets in, particularly at times when painful affects are expressed. As one gets close to a teenager's underlying struggles with sex or aggression, it is important to note whether an ensuing resistance is primarily motivated by the adolescent's anxieties or by the parents' discomfort with newly emerging affects and desires, which are communicated at home.

Earlier, I mentioned Marie, a 16-year-old girl with anorexia nervosa. As Marie began to write letters to an 18-year-old, apparently healthy young man who liked her, she simultaneously reported dreams of having sexual intercourse with this young man and with older men. She suddenly began to miss sessions and indicated her wish to stop treatment. Interpreting the transference elements in her feelings did not dissuade her. She continued to express the feeling that we were wasting time and that she was not getting better fast enough. This was in spite of a twenty-pound weight gain over a period of four and one-half months. Seeing Marie together with her mother and father at this critical point in her treatment was quite revealing and helpful. The father kept looking at Marie with tearful, "basset hound" eyes, saying "I don't mind that you don't want to go camping with me any more; if you are too busy writing to Marty, that's all right! I can always bury myself in work; I have to support you all and send you to college, so that you can see your boyfriend more anyway!" Mother, on the other hand, stated that she was very glad that Marie was now interested in dating, but quickly shifted the subject to an article that she had read in the paper about a coed girl being murdered in a parking lot. She added her convictions that the murderer must have been a sex deviant. It became apparent that the parents needed to be involved in either a parallel conjoint marital therapy or a total family therapy with Marie, to help them all separate out the parental fears and guilt-provoking affects from Marie's own psychosexual internal conflicts.

At times, passive young adolescent boys will be in individual therapy for many months, and will eventually become more assertive and aggressive, both verbally and physically. To the therapist's astonishment, they may suddenly be taken out of treatment by their parents, who are unable to tolerate their new expressions of anger. Seeing such adolescent boys and their parents together, at these moments of resistance, can elicit both the parental anxieties in response to the patient's aggression, as well as those ways in which the teenage boy may be unwittingly provoking his parents by an exaggerated display of his newfound power. An additional problem with such families, particularly in the case of the predelinquent adolescent, lies in confused communication patterns. There may be prohibition of direct expression of aggression at the same time that there is much subtle cueing from the parents provoking antisocial behavior.

Williams (1967a) described how a predelinquent boy was attacked by his parents for investigating areas of the therapist's office that were obviously out of bounds, after they had cued his exploration with their own questions about the restricted area.

The value of seeing the family at these points of resistance is in seeing how the adolescent himself helps start or rekindle the familial anxiety patterns that then act to put down the threatening affects. For example, the adolescent beginning to struggle in individual therapy with his wish to separate from home may in family meetings continue to drop hints about his self-destructive potential once away from his parents. He might state: "Maybe I'd smoke a joint once in a while! Don't worry, I'll find a pad to sleep somewhere." The parents' anxieties are then reawakened in terms of their own reality separation and loss feelings, and in terms of fantasied distortions within them. These intrapsychic distortions may have to do with violence, loss of controls, self-destruction, annihilation, and death, which seem imminent when one separates from parents.

Crises in Families

Series of family meetings aimed at opening up lines of communication can help an adolescent through major points of transitional crisis in a family's life. Crises can be particularly disruptive at points of significant separation, as in divorce, a move to a new neighborhood, a youngster's going away to school, hospitalization, or death. Very often the affects and anxieties that parents feel at times of major crises are repressed only to appear in exaggerated forms within their youngsters. Sudden school phobias or sudden aggressive predelinquent activity frequently occur on the threshold of a divorce or other imminent separation. Also, violent exacerbations of psychosomatic illnesses, such as ulcerative colitis or severe asthma, may occur in an adolescent following the death of a close grandparent or ambivalently loved sibling. Family meetings at such times of crisis allow for an equal sharing of the burden of affect experiences for every member of the family.

With encouragement and selective sharing of his own genuine affects, the therapist can serve as a model to the family to express sadness and rage rather than let them dwell on positive sides of major transitional crises. Parents often emphasize the positive at such times to both reassure their youngsters and to keep repressed their own underlying potential for affect eruption regarding tragic separations.

In preparation for placement of an adolescent outside the home, either in a hospital or in a foster home setting, family meetings can be of great value in bolstering the potential success of the placement. Parents may mask unresolved guilts regarding certain wishes to get rid of a troublesome teenager by resisting a necessary placement. Too, the adolescent may struggle with guilt feelings about leaving his family behind, particularly if there is an unconscious or preconscious awareness of the marital discord that might erupt when the problem teenager is no longer the focus of concern. Such mutual guilts and anxieties, when openly discussed in a series of family meetings, are often worked through and seen in their proper perspective.

The Hospitalized Adolescent

Schween and Gralnick (1965) and others, in their work with hospitalized patients, have during the past few years underlined the necessity for concomitant family therapy while treating the hospitalized patient. The hospitalized adolescent's family particularly needs a family interviewing approach for two reasons. (1) The teenage patient usually returns to the family. (2) Should the therapist see only the designated patient, he is not in a position to consistently deal with the familial resistances to change in the patient. These resistances usually manifest themselves after hospitalization, and alter the gains the adolescent has made by corrective relationships in the hospital milieu. Family meetings while the adolescent is hospitalized permit the therapist and patient to deal with familial, including sibling, resistances to change at every step of the adolescent's gain. The family sessions also help the therapist gauge the optimal therapeutic pace for his adolescent patient with which the family can keep step. This is most important when the plan is for the patient to definitely return to his original family environment.

Recently, a hospitalized, self-destructive, 14-year-old boy made frequent attempts to elope from the hospital, usually after visits from family members. Rather than discontinuing the visiting, family meetings were held on the ward, with the patient, his divorced parents, his mother's fiancé, and his older sister. After several meetings, it became clear to all involved that the patient was acting out the entire family's ambivalence regarding the initial divorce, as well as the mother's imminent remarriage. The patient eventually communicated his loyalty conflicts and his wish for a closer relationship with his estranged father. In addition to the total family meetings, weekly father-son meetings were introduced. The elopement attempts soon subsided.

The Symbiotic Family and Adolescent Identity

For myself, and many of my colleagues, the problem of the locked-in adolescent symbiosis has continued to present a major challenge and therapeutic dilemma. In viewing certain family symbioses, we note a precarious balance between the identity of the adolescent and the diffusion of that identity within the family, within the family identity so to speak. In some families, a family identity is completely lacking; everyone truly "does his own thing." In others, however, the family identity may be so strong as to blot out individual uniqueness. In working with one such family, a professional vaudeville-type stage group, I readily sensed a wholesome family spirit as they discussed with warm feelings their group excitement and pleasures related to traveling around the country together performing as a musical team. However, it took much time and effort to pinpoint any individual, distinct personality differences for the various family members. The parents themselves, as well as the children, frequently confused each other's names, as did the therapist. In that particular family, as well as in one described by Minuchin (1971), the teenager's autonomous identity was lost and submerged by the family's needs. In Minuchin's case, the boy's individuation broke through in the form of an idiosyncratic and life-defying self-starvation, in the symptoms of anorexia nervosa. In the stage family I treated, one of the teenage boy's identity erupted in the form of drug usage and antisocial aggressive acts. Minuchin utilized ongoing family therapy as the primary modality in his treatment. His successful approach to this problem of severe adolescent symbioses led me to reconsider some of my own earlier views (Williams, 1968). I had made a case for the contraindication of family therapy techniques in dealing with some symbiotic adolescents and cited some related negative therapeutic results. I suggested that such families often cooperated with a family treatment approach for long periods of time, just to stay together, paying ear service to but defeating therapeutic insight attempts. Minuchin, however, described a very active involvement by the family therapists in an effort to set up family tasks that highlight the family's internal power plays and eventually force a disruption of the family's pathologic equilibrium. The problem with a passive approach to the locked-in symbiotic family may lie in the probability that the family's homeostatic power is truly stronger than most doctors' therapeutic powers. In the past, my own therapeutic bias regarding the symbiotic adolescent was in the direction of feeling that he desperately needed a separate one-to-one relationship, outside of his family, to encourage his individuation. I believed that in one-to-one therapy, the therapist could demonstrate respect for the adolescent's autonomy, while offering the support necessary to incur trust of relationships outside the cloistered and somewhat paranoid symbiotic family. However, the results of long-term individual therapy with such adolescents, either in hospital or outpatient situations, are often minimal, as are some of the similarly long-term attempts with family therapy. Again, Minuchin emphasized the need for extensive activity by the therapist when working with such families. An example of a therapist-induced family task aimed at highlighting and breaking up control mechanisms within the family is seen in Minuchin's insistence that no one in the family was to eat as long as the anorexic boy would not eat. Since the youngster was already secretly in control of his entire family, with the symptom of anorexia, and since the parents were already helpless, the family task merely brought to the surface and underscored that the boy was truly the despot. The despot interpretation, and family-fasting task, led to all kinds of severe familial disruptions. The therapist had to be available day and night during the ensuing crisis to move in and encourage the forward movement and individuation at the point of crisis.

In certain families, teenage boys or girls "will not permit" their parents to go away without them to parties or on vacations. In exploring the value of family therapy and family tasks with such families, I have introduced the task of insisting that the parents go out, after many sessions of dealing with both the adolescent's and parents' resistances to such individuation and freedom. My experiences in this regard are similar to those of Minuchin in relation to the essentiality of therapist availability for crisis intervention. For example, when in response to the parents' first weekend away a teenage boy crashes his car, or a teenage girl makes a manipulative but dangerous suicide attempt, the therapist has to be ready to continue to push for the separation, while making himself and appropriate others available to the adolescent for physical and emotional help.

For the present I feel that a combined approach that utilizes individual treatment, series of family meetings, and major attention to encouraging peer relationships is necessary in dealing with the symbiotic adolescent and his family.

CONCLUSIONS

As therapists, but primarily as human beings, we like to know our own roles and identity, with a minimum of confusion. Psychotherapy with adolescents can be overwhelming for the therapist because of complicating family forces, peer crises, legal entanglements, the pressure for guidance, and direct advice. We may wish the adolescent to go elsewhere. On the other hand, we may handle our frustration by magnifying the value of confidentiality and, with our adolescent patient, "hide from the world." This unfortunate overemphasis on confidentiality can at times constrict the therapist's diagnostic vision, as well as foreclose an opportunity to utilize family interviewing techniques, a most helpful treatment modality when working with adolescents.

Family therapy offers a means to overcome resistance to an adolescent's psychosocial and psychosexual development. For some adolescent problems the family approach should be the primary therapeutic modality. In family sessions, the therapist can offer a point of view and an attitude that embodies respect for the individuation of the adolescent, as well as respect for the family group and its identity. He can encourage communication of affects and the expression of feelings of intimacy in ways which do not threaten regression to infantile or erotic ties. My overall recommendation is geared toward a flexible approach, which includes family and individual therapy, and which permits direct observation of those dynamic familial interpersonal forces impinging on the adolescent's psyche.

Flexibility of approach encompasses many considerations: When do we involve the entire family in a regular ongoing treatment? When do we utilize one or a series of meetings for diagnostic purposes? Will family therapy help individuation or promote continued symbioses in certain symbiotic families?

Teachers and students of adolescent psychiatry need much greater exposure to family techniques if we are to acquire significant clinical wisdom regarding these questions.

One can feel overwhelmed by the chaos of an adolescent's intrapsychic life. One can feel still further overwhelmed when seeing an adolescent together with his family, in the same room, over long periods of time. Nonetheless, I feel that we need to expose students of adolescent psychiatry to the reality of these interdigitating, overwhelming forces. More so than with any other age group, the psyche of the adolescent cannot be undertood without appreciating the impinging and shifting pressures of the familial field.

REFERENCES

Brown, S. L. (1964). Clinical impression of the impact of family group interviewing on child and adolescent psychiatric practice. *Journal of the American Academy of Child Psychiatry*, 3, 5, 688-696.

Brown, S. L. (1969). Diagnosis, clinical management and family interviewing. In *Science and Psychoanalysis*, Vol. 14, J. Masserman, ed. New York: Grune & Stratton.

Brown, S. L. (1970). Family for adolescents. *Psychiatric Opinion*, 7, 1.

Minuchin, S. (1971). Re-conceptualization of adolescent dynamics from the family point of view. In *Teaching and Learning Adolescent Psychiatry*, D. Offer and J. F. Masterson, eds. Springfield, Ill.: Charles C Thomas.

Paul, N. L., and Grosser, G. H. (1965. Operational mourning and its role in conjoint family therapy. *Community Mental Health Journal*, 1, 4:339-345.

Schween, P. H., and Gralnick, A. (1965). Factors affecting family therapy in the hospital setting. *Comprehensive Psychiatry*, 7, 5, 424-431.

Williams, F. S. (1967a). Family interviews for diagnostic evaluations in child psychiatry. Paper presented to the American Orthopsychiatric Association, New York City.

Williams, F. S. (1967b). Family therapy: A critical assessment. *American Journal of Orthopsychiatry*, 37, 5, 912-919.

Williams, F. S. (1968). Family therapy. In *Modern Psychoanalysis*. J. Marmor, ed. Pp. 387-406. New York: Basic Books.

Williams, F. S. (1970). Alienation of youth as reflected in the hippie movement. *Journal of the American Academy of Child Psychiatry*, 9, 2, 251-263.

Wynne, L. C. (1965). Some indications and contraindications for exploration of family therapy. In *Intensive Family Therapy*, I. Boszormenyi-Nagy and J. L. Framo, eds. Pp. 289-322. New York: Harper & Row.

12

Family Therapy with Adolescents and the Process of Intergenerational Reconciliation

HELM STIERLIN, M.D., Ph.D.

The adolescent who attempts to separate himself from his family faces three interdependent tasks. All these tasks bear on his psychological growth. They relate to his individuation as well as to his (relative) separation.

I would like to define these tasks as *tasks of reconciliation*. Various aspects of them have been described in the psychiatric and psychoanalytic literature, particularly in the works of A. Freud (1946), P. Blos (1962, 1970), and E. H. Erikson (1950, 1959, 1968). By emphasizing their reconciling nature we can, I believe, best study their individual, as well as family system, aspects and trace their implications for family therapy.

The first of these tasks of reconciliation refers to the psychophysiologic differentiations and integrations which are required of the adolescent. We may speak here, for lack of better wording, of the *task of integrative reconciliation*. This task encompasses the differentiation of the adolescent's drives, feelings and motivations and their integration into a viable organization of defenses and identity. This task is made difficult by the powerful, partly hormonally-caused upsurges of his sexual and aggressive energies, which find few, if any, acceptable outlets. These energies, while pressuring for discharge, must be absorbed into and tamed by a structured

Revised version of a paper presented at a Symposium, "Community and Family Psychiatry: Experiences, Assessment and Problems of Evaluation," at the Institute of Community and Family Psychiatry, Department of Psychiatry, Jewish General Hospital, Montreal, P. Q., Canada, October 10 and 11, 1969.

identity that should be as solid as it should be differentiated and complex. This applies particularly to his (or her) gender identity.

The second task presupposes such a framework but also transcends it. In my book, *Conflict and Reconciliation* (1969), I have tried to adumbrate this task which I would now like to call the *task of adaptive reconciliation*. This task demands that modern adolescents—more, I believe, than members of any other age group—must reconcile several action trends or "existential" attitudes, which are interrelated, yet polarized. Most important here are the polarities "doing—undergoing," "choice—renunciation," and "self-realization—self-limiting."

"Doing," as here conceived, refers to the adolescent's needs for self-affirmation and self-determination. It stands for his ability and willingness to experience himself as the shaper of his destiny, as a center of self-initiated action, of responsibility and executive power. It implies that he can say and feel: "I do, I plan for myself, I am my maker, I am responsible for myself."

The adolescent must reconcile such doing with undergoing, referring to his ability and willingness to experience his actions as influenced and/or determined by forces outside himself. It implies that he can recognize and accept the "givens" of this world, and himself as one of these givens. It implies that he can say and feel: "I undergo, I depend on others, I cannot totally plan myself, I am not absolutely responsible."

For the adolescent who grows up in our changing and complex society, the above dialectic becomes radicalized. He must be more undergoing than previous generations in the sense that he, in order to live successfully in this society, must open himself up to wide-ranging sources of learning and, along therewith, must remain excessively dependent on those bodies which facilitate such learning—mainly the universities and the parents who pay his tuition. At the same time, he is strongly pressured into "doing" and "self-determination" in the sense that he must, in the words of Erikson, make "a series of ever-narrowing selections of personal, occupational, sexual and ideological commitments." He is thus pressured to make choices and to achieve renunciations. In so doing, he must realize himself by limiting himself, or—expressed slightly differently—he must choose to realize himself by establishing and accepting his limits.

This adolescent must, next, attempt to liquidate the burden he carries from his interpersonal past. He must, this means, try to correct and outgrow those fixations, traumata, and consequences of an uneven development which were forced upon him by others and which now threaten to hamper his future growth. He must, further, try to get rid of, or at least modify, those bad parental inner objects (or object images) that might thwart his object relations to come.

The *task of reparative reconciliation,* the third interdependent task mentioned above, encompasses all these attempts. If these are to be successful they demand not seldom a "reintegration at the base," characterized by inner turmoil, intense anxiety, and a temporary disintegration and regressive loosening of the personality. Also, these attempts imply a painful mourning process, as recently described by M. Sugar (1968), through which the adolescent disengages himself at least partly from his parents qua inner objects (this is often referred to as his separation from his oedipal parents) and qua real persons. Finally, I include in the task of reparative reconciliation the possible coming to grips with the above burden through artistic creativity. This avenue, though, seems open only to a limited number of adolescents.

RECONCILIATION ON THE FAMILY LEVEL

These three tasks of reconciliation, in order to be understood and supported by our professional help, must now be seen in a family context. When focusing on the family, we deal with a different system, a different order of complexity, and a different level of reconciliation. We realize that, in the words of the philosopher Hegel (1805), "the doing of one is the doing of others," or, more specifically, the growth of one is the growth of others, or the separation of one is the separation of others. The others are here, of course, chiefly the parents of the adolescent and, to some extent, his siblings.

Let me turn to the family system by taking up, one after the other, the three tasks of reconciliation, as outlined above. I shall examine how these three tasks imply a reconciling effort on the family level. Thereafter I shall consider how the family therapist may assist such effort on this level.

In taking up the first task—which I called the *task of integrative reconciliation*—I shall limit myself to discussing some problems which are posed by the adolescent's awakening sexuality and his (or her) need to achieve a viable gender identity.

With regard to this problem area we can state the following general rule: an adolescent can accept and master his budding sexuality only to the extent that his or her parents have done so with respect to their own sexuality. In order to illustrate this point (and others to be taken up later), I shall now take recourse to a family whom I shall call the Allen family, consisting of Mr. and Mrs. Allen, two respectable middle-class suburbanites, and Evelyn, their only daughter.

The Allens came for treatment at the Family Studies Section of the Adult Psychiatry Branch, National Institute of Mental Health, because Evelyn, a sweet looking and somewhat precocious girl of sixteen and a half, had run into the kind of troubles that seem nowadays almost standard. She had taken to drugs (acid, speed, pot and others) and bad boys (usually two or three at a time). Also, she had become truant, and, in order to cover up her truancy, had entangled herself in a web of lies, deceptions and forgings of passes. Getting more and more into a panic, Evelyn had finally run away to New York where, after several days, she was rescued by her devastated father. Evelyn believed at that time she was pregnant and was tormented by fears that she might give birth to a LSD-deformed monster. (She was not pregnant.)

In the family sessions Evelyn found little parental understanding or even sympathy for her agonies. Instead, the parents appeared to compound Evelyn's sexual difficulties. The mother alternated chiefly between stances of righteous indignation and an (to the observer) insatiable, though covertly expressed, interest in Evelyn's unsavory company and sexual experiences. The father, through sly (though barely noticeable) "come-on" smiles, encouraged Evelyn to put her dumb mother into place, thereby intensifying the oedipal tangle and preventing its resolution. Evelyn responded to the father's messages and exasperated her mother by being defiant and cocksure. She (Evelyn), with almost sadistic glee, would now present herself as a real swinger, as somebody who was "with it," whereas her mother—"this most pathetic example of someone over thirty"—was out of everything, just a stupid, hopeless square.

In the family therapy it became quickly apparent how the parents' own sexual difficulties bore on Evelyn's plight. The mother, a flamboyant yet frigid, hysterical woman, channeled into Evelyn that mixture of prurient sexual excitability and righteous moralizing which had become the chief manifestation of, as well as coping device for, her own sexual immaturity and conflictfulness. The father, an overcontrolled, obsessive type, behaved rejectingly as well as seductively vis-à-vis Evelyn. The latter, subjected to confusing messages, had responded by developing her confused "hit and run sexuality."

Evelyn, it follows from these considerations, in order to achieve a viable and mature sexual identity of her own, required her parents to do likewise. She put the latter under pressure to work on their own growth and to make certain reconciling moves. We will better understand what this implied for the parents when we consider, now, within the family context, the second task mentioned above—the one which I have called the *task of adaptive reconciliation*. In turning to this task, we deal with a problem area that encompasses what traditionally has come to be known as the adolescent's *quest for autonomy*.

I indicated earlier that this second task of reconciliation tends to become radicalized for the modern adolescent due to the growing and conflicting social pressures he has to meet. This radicalization, I believe, is also reflected on the family level. We notice here how such radicalization affects and highlights certain areas of conflict and of needed reconciliation within the family. Let me, to make this clearer, again turn to the Allens.

I have already mentioned Evelyn's rebellious defiance of her mother, as when she called the latter "a hopeless square over thirty." I must now add that Evelyn had generalized this defiance into a rejection of almost everything that her parents considered good and worthwhile. In this respect Evelyn differed little from many other members of her age group. Not only did Evelyn flaunt a four-letter vocabulary, dress sloppily and in hippie fashion, experiment liberally with drugs and, it seemed, sleep with every boy in sight, but she also wrote—as editor of her high school paper—articles in praise of Castro and Ho Chi Minh and plotted, with the help of some "SDS advisers," the ouster of her "reactionary" high school superintendent. In the light of such generalized, as well as radicalized, rebellion on Evelyn's part, we can better understand why her parents found it difficult to be patient and sympathetic with her. Pushed into a corner and feeling threatened in what they believed and valued most, they could, it seemed, no longer afford understanding or sympathy. Instead, they could only experience rage and exasperation. And in experiencing these painful emotions, they sensed that all meaningful communication between them and their daughter had broken down.

Anybody who in these days has worked on an adolescent ward can probably empathize with Evelyn's parents—he knows what it feels like to be constantly shown up as wrong, "square," worthless and impotent. And so can, in fact, many a parent, teacher or citizen over thirty who sees modern youth picking on and espousing with seeming devilish cunning every possible hero or value that runs counter to his or her own cherished beliefs—pitting Che Guevara and John Lennon against the "Establishment," or the hippie life in the "here and now" against the plastic, rat-race culture of suburbia.

We can speak here of the adolescent's *self-determination against his parents.* Such self-determination has always been part of the conflict of generations and of the separation drama of adolescence. And it has always tended to become fiercer, the stronger the underlying emotional ties have been. I believe, however, that today many an adolscent's self-determination against his own parents has—for reasons which I cannot elaborate—tended to become more radical, as well as mandatory, than in previous times. Along therewith, it has necessitated balancing moves—on the part of the adolescent and of the parents—of corresponding strength.

Such radicalized self-determination, in order not to result in mere intergenerational warfare, must now include a self-determination *with* the parents, that is, it must imply an ability and willingness in all partners to keep the dialogue going—despite temporary alienations and breakdowns in communication. Doing and self-determination, this means, have to be reconciled with undergoing and receptivity. And this reconciliation must reflect a family effort. A family climate and culture must be created and maintained wherein mutual—intergenerational!—learning and mutual growth may occur along with mutual individuation and separation.

I see it here—and this brings me to the issue of family therapy—as the main task of the family therapist to help create and improve such family climate and culture—and to do so in the face of the powerful forces which threaten to erode or overthrow the latter. In trying to resolve this task he will with profit reflect on the concept of a shared focus of attention, as elaborated by L. C. Wynne. Wynne, in collaboration with M. T. Singer, has made this the pivotal concept for the study and classification of relational pathology in families with schizophrenic offspring (Wynne and Singer, 1963a, b; Singer and Wynne, 1965a, b). It becomes pivotal also, I believe, when applied to the study of, and psychotherapeutic intervention in, the separation drama of (neurotic and relatively normal) adolescents. By our pointing out, again and again, how the parents and their adolescent offspring fail to share such a common focus, how they avoid listening to each other, and how they cannot confirm either agreement or disagreement, we establish ourselves as facilitators of communication instead of the stern, guilt-inducing and partial judges they expect us to be. We become the chief reconciling agents.

In the case of the Allens, our chosen example, the psychotherapists had to persistently take up the many ways in which the family members tended to talk parallel to and against, but not with, each other. In thus serving as facilitators of family communication, the therapists not only helped to de-radicalize the bitter intergenerational (and marital) war, but they also made it possible for each member to gain new perspectives through and about the other members, that is, to learn from and about one another. Such learning to learn, made possible within a seemingly immobilized family, could then lead to further needed changes. These changes, in order to be beneficial, had to occur in the area of the parents' own thwarted sexual development, as mentioned earlier. But along with and beyond that, these changes had to encompass growth on what appears to be an even deeper level. It is this level to which I turn next.

This level relates to the third reconciling task mentioned in the beginning—the *task of reparative reconciliation.* This task I described as being aimed at correcting and outgrowing the burden of one's past. Let us now consider how this third task becomes a task for the whole family and how it affects our needed psychotherapeutic interventions.

Again, one aspect of the Allen family may serve as an illustration. As the therapy with them got underway, I began to notice the following characteristic sequence unfolding between the mother and Evelyn. They both seemed to become repeatedly sad and grief-stricken and then doubly vituperative with each other. When I encouraged them to put their sadness and grief into words, Evelyn talked in a vague way about feeling lonely and bad, whereas the mother turned more and more to talking about her past, about her own parents, and about her own unhappy youth. In so doing, she related the following. The daughter of poor European immigrants, she, the mother, had had to endure her mother's constant nagging tirades, had been overwhelmed and overburdened with household chores, and had been forbidden to take part in the "frivolous" activities of her peers. Among these peers was a cousin, Erna, a beautiful, outgoing and popular girl whom she envied and tried to emulate. This cousin Erna came to stand in Mrs. Allen's mind for all that which she, as an adolescent, could not be and could not have. As Mrs. Allen talked about this cousin she emphasized how much Evelyn resembled her, and at one point she inadvertently called her daughter Erna.

It seemed now significant that the mother, after having told of her deprivation at the hands of her own mother, appeared to turn against Evelyn with a vengeance, victimizing her mercilessly. But it seemed no less significant that Evelyn, by some particularly defiant and provocative word or gesture, appeared to actively invite such victimization. How can we explain this?

I am, above all, indebted to I. Boszormenyi-Nagy (1972; Boszormenyi-Nagy and Spark, 1973) for understanding more fully the meaning of a transactional sequence such as the one just outlined. This sequence reveals some crucial features and problems in the mother's and Evelyn's efforts at a reparative reconciliation, as I understand this concept. Risking the danger of oversimplification, we may state these features and problems as follows:

After having learned to communicate more freely with Evelyn, the mother began to see the latter a little differently. She seemed to become more able to perceive of Evelyn as a person in her own right. Along with thus viewing Evelyn more objectively, she could, with the support of the therapists, face and experience some of the deprivation and frustration she had suffered at the hands of her own mother. This led to her becoming depressed and grief-stricken, as indicated above. But also—and this seems important—it caused an upsurge of painful guilt. Dimly the mother seemed to grow aware that through all these years she had tried to take Evelyn to account for what her own mother had done to her, that she had turned Evelyn into a projection screen and externalized prop for her coming to grips with her own unresolved conflicts and seemingly unendurable frustrations, as these related to her own mother.

In addition to thus casting Evelyn, in important respects, into the role of her own mother (that is, parentifying Evelyn), she had also attributed to her daughter many qualities of her cousin Erna, the emulated idol of her own adolescence. Thus, Mrs. Allen brought further conflicting pressures to bear on Evelyn. She covertly encouraged Evelyn to reenact Erna's wild adolescent sprees and to thereby provide her, the mother, with vicarious thrills. At the same time, she castigated Evelyn for being wild, promiscuous and irresponsible, spicing such castigation with all the envious hatred she had felt—and still felt—for Erna.

In beginning to experience grief and sadness, the mother started to work on her reparative reconciliation, facilitating thereby her own and Evelyn's liberation from the burdens of their past. And this process had to be mutual. Evelyn, also, we noticed, began to appear sad and grief-stricken and Evelyn, also, we can assume, had started to reappraise her mother. But why, we must ask, was the work of repair and grief punctuated by the earlier-mentioned relapses into the bitter game of defiance and victimization?

These relapses, I believe, become understandable when one is cognizant of the massive guilt which began to pervade the mother's—and Evelyn's— awareness. To the extent that the mother could start to see Evelyn as a person in her own right and that she began to undertake long overdue repairs in relation to her daughter, she could not help becoming more conscious of what she had done to Evelyn—hence the onrush of guilt which superimposed more pain on the pain she already felt. It was in an attempt to cope with this guilt and its pain, I believe, that the mother turned again into a ruthless victimizer. And it was, I believe further, in an attempt to assuage the mother's guilt and pain that Evelyn, by being outrageously provocative, offered herself to be victimized. We may speak of a collusion between the mother and daughter in the service of a mutual assuagement of guilt, a process which has been thoroughly described by I. Boszormenyi-Nagy (1972).

I consider it one of the central tasks of family therapy to break up such collusion in the service of guilt assuagement and to thereby facilitate each family member's reparative reconciliations.

This, then, finally brings into focus the system aspect of the family interaction. This system aspect, as it relates to the issue under discussion, has already been adumbrated by Hegel in *The Phenomenology of the Spirit* (written in 1805). Herein Hegel made the relationship between master and servant (*Herr und Knecht*) the paradigm of a relationship between two unequals, of which one presents himself as the powerful victimizer and the other as the weak victim. This relationship, Hegel pointed out, tends to create a dialectic momentum through which the victimizer loses and the victim gains psychological power. The more the master has to rely on the servant for making his (the master's) life productive and meaningful, the more he becomes psychologically dependent on and governed by the latter. The victim, in other words, becomes more powerful, as he lets himself be more victimized.

Translated into modern family dynamics, this means that the victimized adolescent usually becomes the most powerful family member because he is in the best position to operate the guilt lever. It means also that he, in order to spare himself the painful work of separation and growth, will tend to either provoke or hold onto his victimization. And it means, further, that the therapist, in order to break up the above-described collusion and to facilitate a reparative reconciliation in all concerned, must erode the victim's powers for inducing guilt. He must interpret the victim's masochism, that is, his enjoyment of suffering, and the sadism which is therein implied. (Such masochism presents the most difficult technical problem in the psychoanalysis of individual patients, just as it does in family therapy.)

In the case of the Allens this meant, above all, that the provocative and, yet, underhandedly masochistic and controlling elements in Evelyn's behavior had to become analyzed before the parents could make substantial progress in their own task of reparative reconciliation. We recognize here one of the paradoxes with which family therapy constantly confronts us: in order to help Evelyn in her separation *from,* and self-determination *against,* her parents, the therapists seemingly had to align themselves with the parents against the hapless Evelyn. (I emphasize the word *seemingly,* because the analysis of Evelyn's wielding of power through the enjoyment of her victimization represents at best a "dialectical" sort of alignment.) In so doing, they helped to undermine the total family system wherein victimizer and victim appeared inexorably bound to each other and where, in such mutual bondage, real individual growth and separation had become impossible for all.

If we look back on how our exposition of the adolescent's and his family's separation drama unfolded, we notice how our awareness of the problems and of the necessary therapeutic interventions shifted. At first the adolescent's plight, as conventionally described in the psychoanalytic and psychiatric literature, came into view. In then considering the family context we saw how the parents, on account of their own immaturities and unresolved conflicts, had given rise to this plight and tended to prolong it. Yet, when we asked how we should deal with the parents, our focus shifted again to the adolescent as the one who exerted the most powerful guilt leverage. From there we could support the parents in their grief work which only then had become possible. And so, I believe, it has to go on—in a complex dialectical process of shifting foci, a process which, hopefully, leads to an ever expanding awareness and growth, on the part of the family members *and* on the part of the family therapists, and which reflects successful reconciliation on all the three levels outlined above.

REFERENCES

BLOS, P. (1962). *On Adolescence: A Psychoanalytic Interpretation.* New York: Free Press of Glencoe.
BLOS, P. (1970). *The Young Adolescent: Clinical Studies.* New York: Free Press.
BOSZORMENYI-NAGY, I. (1972). Loyalty implications of the transference model in psychotherapy. *Archives of General Psychiatry,* 27:374-380.
BOSZORMENYI-NAGY, L., and SPARK, G. (1973). *Invisible Loyalties.* New York: Harper and Row.
ERIKSON, E. H. (1950). *Childhood and Society.* New York: Norton.
ERIKSON, E. H. (1959). *Identity and the Life Cycle.* New York: International Universities Press.
ERIKSON, E. H. (1968). *Identity, Youth and Crisis.* New York: Norton.
FREUD, A. (1946). *The Ego and the Mechanisms of Defense.* New York: International Universities Press.

HEGEL, G. (1910). *The Phenomenology of the Spirit* (1805), 2 Vols., Translated by
J. B. Baillie. London: Swann Sonnenschein.
SINGER, M. T., and WYNNE, L. C. (1965a). Thought disorder and family relations of
schizophrenics. III. Methodology using projective techniques. *Archives of General
Psychiatry,* 12:187-200.
SINGER, M. T., and WYNNE, L. C. (1965b). Thought disorder and family relations of
schizophrenics. IV. Results and implications. *Archives of General Psychiatry,* 12:
201-212.
STIERLIN, H. (1969). *Conflict and Reconciliation.* New York: Doubleday, and Anchor
Science House.
SUGAR, M. (1968). Normal adolescent mourning. *American Journal of Psychotherapy,*
22:258-269.
WYNNE, L. C., and SINGER, M. T. (1963a). Thought disorder and family relations of
schizophrenics. I. A research strategy. *Archives of General Psychiatry,* 9:191-198.
WYNNE, L. C., and SINGER, M. T. (1963b). Thought disorder and family relations of
schizophrenics. II. A classification of forms of thinking. *Archives of General
Psychiatry,* 9:199-206.

13

The Symptomatic Adolescent – An AWOL Family Member

CARL A. WHITAKER, M.D.

Treatment of the adolescent is often considered to lay midway between play therapy for children and individual analytic treatment for adults. During the 50's adolescent psychotherapy was chaotic because we couldn't handle the adolescent's profound ambivalence: one moment he yearned to be dependent, and the next resented his dependence on the therapist. At a later moment, he'd fight for his independence and resent the therapist for not activating that freedom. However, by 1960, techniques of treating the adolescent with kid gloves had made individual treatment of the adolescent a fairly successful procedure. Therapists sophisticated in the use of psychotherapy could define the interpersonal distance the individual adolescent tolerated and thus leave him free to move closer as he needed intimacy and away as he needed separateness. Thus, neither the bind of all-out dependency nor the specter of rejection destroyed the therapeutic movement.

The transference-countertransference phenomena in the treatment of the 1970's adolescent, however, are uniquely complex. The contemporary therapist is stuck with not only the natural ambivalence but also the reality of the new cultural gap and its problems. The adolescent patient feels humiliated asking for help from an adult who belongs to the "establishment" and he is thereby uptight about being in therapy. He has also been conditioned by the peer group to believe that having any relationship to the older generation is disloyal to the group and denotes infantile hang-ups. However, his chance of getting help from his peers is also very restricted. Peers as social growth facilitators are empathetic only to a limited degree and only if the stress is in the direction of the accepted social role structure. Bitter anger at parents can be shared, but depression or strange behavior may be alienating. Creative therapists, however, have learned how to bridge the generation gap by their own therapeutic youth and by a capacity to hang loose in the therapeutic relationship. Some employ the music, the new language and the mores of the teenage component of our society as a communication bridge.

During the World Congress of Psychiatry in Mexico in 1971, I was horrified to sit through a half day of papers on treatment of adolescent patients with no consideration given to the use of family therapy. Transference resolution was apparently the only method accepted. May I suggest family therapy as a modality for the treatment of *every* adolescent patient?

Although the adolescent seeking treatment is obviously an individual and is clearly suffering from intrapsychic stress, that does not mean that the only methodology for treatment is individual therapy. Being a good physician does not mean putting salve on every wound and often individual treatment of the most concerned and expert quality is like a shot of morphine for the pain of appendicitis. It does not resolve the problem but makes the situation more serious by obscuring the systems component of the presenting symptom.

Freud's devotion to research on the adult and his intrapsychic stress has delayed our perception of the total context of individual stress. This is nowhere more evident than in treatment of the adolescent and his heartache. The usual symptomatic adolescent is an individual who has broken with his family in a precipitous, painful and unsatisfactory manner. Both he and the family are bleeding from the wounds of this operation. Often dropping out at such an early emotional age results in a more profound dependence and unresolvable ambivalence in the escapee and in the family system as well. If you accept this conception, then the treatment of adolescents is really a reentry problem and a debriefing problem. The adolescent is really a family dropout who has not stayed through his senior year, the year in which he would gain pre-adult status and which is ended by a graduation ceremony. He needs to reenter the family system and separate to try life on his own. This then would not follow the divorce model referred to above, but make possible a group membership, free of enslavement on either side of the generation gap.

It has been hypothesized that one need not have stress during adolescence and that it is possible to leave the family in a ceremonial, constructive and mutually satisfying manner. This was graphically expressed by an adult graduate student involved in couples therapy. She had spent a year in psychotherapy with her husband in an effort to prevent a legalized siamese twin operation to divorce the two of them. The therapist remarked towards the end of therapy how good it would be to not have to see them anymore. She said, in surprise, "I wish to hell my father and mother had said that just once. I could have left without feeling so guilty." She did work through in the transference the reentry and graduation from this therapy family, but yearned to do the same with her family of origin. Needless to say, marital therapy is not a very economical system for reentering and graduating from the family of origin.

What are the indications and contraindications for family treatment? This author is convinced that there are no contraindications *if* the family is available and if the therapist is willing to struggle with the whole unit. This is probably true whether the identified patient is an adolescent or an adult but is certainly most obvious in the treatment of the adolescent. The family is *the* controlling agent in any adolescent's life—far out of proportion to time spent with them, and in spite of physical distance.

Although the family in treatment may include only adoptive or foster parents or may have only a mother in economic privation and battle fatigue from child-care, the family therapy must deal with the intrapsychic family who determine many of the dynamics of therapy. The alcoholic father who left ten years before may be a most authentic ghost for the teenager and for his mother. The addition of the probation worker or the school counselor to the family therapy team may not only be helpful, but may also teach the parent figures a greater flexibility and the therapist new aspects of his professional job.

One adult of 45 years atempted suicide at the exact age his father did. A mother phones her married daughter in midweek and a single remark ruins the rest of the week. A daughter (of 35 years) acts out periodically in order to reconnect with her parents. These recurrent life stories emphasize the power of the family. Therapists, then, the cultural surrogates, must develop a method for filling the gap left by the decay of the traditional puberty rites that made the transition from childhood to adulthood a victory over dependence and an inauguration into the adult world (Flescher, 1968).

J. D. was a 19-year-old student who had been diagnosed as manic psychotic by a university inpatient service in a different city and put on lithium and stelazine. He had moved from city to city making repeated individual therapy contracts and then breaking them. He had stopped his lithium, as well as other medications, and had stopped his psychotherapy. Finally one therapist asked for a conference with mother, father and sister. In the middle of this four-hour conference, he challenged the mother on her chaos and she then, for the first time, explained to her 19-year-old son about her five years of psychotherapy beginning when he was three, and how she had lied to her own mother by saying that these appointments five times a week for five years were dental treatment. Father went on then to explain that it was not his life of pure scientific research that left no time or affect to relate to his son. It was really a life filled with nights of panic during those years when mother was in psychotherapy and during J.D.'s recent mental hospital periods. Since J.D. was eight, Dad had been fighting to keep mother's secret and to protect her from all stress, lest she become emotionally sick again. He was, of course, also trying to protect her from the shame of this confession. The son's response to this was startling. "So Dad, that's why you always raised hell with me whenever I tried to stand up for myself against mother. I never knew before that you really gave a damn about me or mother and I have never seen you cry before in my life. What a flip this is."

Episodes like this make one wonder whether there is much hope of resolving this kind of affective chaos by even long-term individual transference work. I am tempted to, but will not, quote Jim Framo who says, "One hug from the mother is worth a thousand hugs from the therapist."

Bill's mother phoned from a nearby city. "It's my 18-year-old son. His therapist has given up after seeing him for four years and told me to call you."—"Sorry, I only see families."—"You mean you won't see him?"—"I only see families."—"All right, I'll come then."— "What about father?"—"That's one of the problems. We're getting a divorce."—"Sorry, better find somebody else."—"Okay, I'll bring him."—"Who do you live with now?"—"My mother and father."— "Bring them too."—"That's crazy. They don't have anything to do with my son."—"Sorry then, find somebody else."—"Okay, I'll bring them."—"How about your husband's parents?"—"They live 500 miles away."—"Well, have him call me if he can't get them to come." Everybody showed up except father's mother who had a sudden attack of rheumatism. The conference was scheduled for three hours and as is my custom, I started asking father's father my standard question, "What's going on in the family?" I then went to mother's father, mother's mother, then to father, then to mother. During a solid hour, I got nothing except the pseudomutual line, "All is fine. We're a close family. We don't understand why this boy became upset." Finally, I got to the identified patient—"Listen, this whole family sounds crazy. Nobody can see past the end of his nose. Everybody thinks the family is perfect and yet you're accused of being crazy for four years." Bill, the diagnosed schizophrenic, then said, "Oh, I can tell you what's wrong. My father's father is the younger brother of my mother's mother and 'big sister' has been telling 'little brother' what to do ever since she was five. I'm the victim of a three generation family war, and all my life I have been trained to be a Hasidic scholar and I don't know how to get out of the corner I'm in."

Part of his difficulty was the usual child and adolescent dedication to helping the parents make a better life. It's hard to know how much of his emotional distress was psychological and how much familial, but it seems fairly clear that individual psychotherapy was not going to do much to this three generational imprint. The identified patient was a victim of a war between forces much greater than he himself could control.

Sue was 20 and quite clearly suffering from a psychotic break. The family was called in, including three married siblings, all of whom lived in a neighboring state. Mother and father gave the story of a close, friendly, warm family. Everybody got along well together and nobody had any idea why Sue was upset. After a half hour of this one of the adult sisters said, "Dad, I don't understand why you go on like this. Sue doesn't know anything about her own family. Mother was in a mental hospital for six months. I've been in psychotherapy for three years. My sister's been in psychotherapy for four years and she's still in treatment. My brother has just begun. Why don't you tell the doctor?" With this type of programmed family secret, how could Sue expect to grow? The honesty of an intimate, loving family with open communication was unknown. The family consultation thus enabled Sue to get some sense that she was not the black sheep of the family and allowed mother and father to at least have the honor of facing life the way it was and of expressing their anxiety and concern in some better way than by hiding it.

The identified patient is many times only the top of the iceberg and the symptom that brings one patient to the therapist may well represent a state of family chaos which should be treated as a whole family pattern of pain and distress. The family symptom may be intrapsychic to one scapegoat or several. It may be concurrent in several family members or appear in a serial progression. The system controls the functions of its component members. Therapy often changes the components but still need not alter the system itself (Whitaker and Miller, 1969).

Bill brought his wife to the therapist because she was a serious alcoholic. It was revealed two interviews later that Bill also collects art prints. He has 35,000 prints piled in various places in their small house. Some weeks later their pompous, effeminate ten-year-old, who quite dominated the family, was discovered to be suffering from a school phobia. The school counselor was invited into the therapy then and two weeks later he discovered that, for the past six months, the 17-year-old son had been leaving as though for school each morning on schedule but had never shown up at school. The school had never registered him. The family seemed such a caricature that I suggested to the 15-year-old son that the least he could do would be to steal a car so he could belong to the family. That broke the family into a freedom to laugh at themselves. What if I had tried to treat the ten-year-old in individual therapy for the school phobia, or mother for her alcoholism, or father for his compulsive collecting? Any one of them could have been in individual therapy for years.

If an adolescent leaves his family in a self-induced puberty ceremony of rebellion, if he breaks with the family without some group resolution of the problems of the symbiosis amongst them, if he leaves without joining in an overt family effort to resolve his desertion—rather than by a therapeutic effort to relieve the individual and group stress—he is stuck with guilt and not free to instigate a new and creative life. He may then be compelled to reconstruct the old family again, to work out that senior year and that graduation ceremony at work, at play or in his marriage.

Why does individual therapy work at all? Many times it seems individual therapy works because this patient and this therapist and their transference power are enough so that the patient can change the dynamics of his entire family. It may even be that the effects of individual therapy are only lasting if family change is possible. If one-to-one therapy is not powerful enough to change the family, then individual treatment fails to individuate the patient or to help him break with his family of origin. Such failure also establishes a wall between the patient and his family.

If the individual therapy transference relationship as a symbolic illusion becomes defined as the only acceptable pattern for parent-child relationships, then, of course, the actual family of origin can never live up to that all-loving delusion. The patient then tends to establish geographic or psychological distance and to maintain the illusion of adulthood while he carries on a covert effort to return to his momma for the graduation ceremony that never happened, or he develops other relationships which are substitutes for the family. The most conspicuous of these, of course, is marriage.

Family conferences may also serve as a basis for useful interaction with the disturbed teenagers. Not all that is useful is symbolic.

Mary, a 17-year-old freshman in college was three months into family treatment after referral due to "loss of ego-boundaries." Sunday at 7:00 A.M. she phoned the author. "Dr. W., my father won't let me do anything. Wouldn't let me do my thing. I wanted popcorn last night and I didn't have any at my apartment so I came home to make it. I stayed overnight and this morning they won't leave me alone. They keep coming after me." *Therapist*: "You came after them last night. Why don't you go back to your apartment?"—"Hey, that's a good idea. I just will do that. Say, another thing, will you teach me how to be real?"—"I'll try."—"Okay, thanks. Good-bye."

It's pretty clear that the next time the family gets together there is going to be a pretty good-sized family fight. Since closeness and separation between adolescents and the family group increase point and counterpoint, the sense of we-ness and individuation for Mary and her family and its five individual members will increase slightly because Mary, first, ached for love enough to go home for popcorn and, then, dared her loneliness enough to leave the family next morning for her apartment. Could the same little jiggle from the therapist have had the same effect in individual therapy? Probably, but I'll bet the change would be more liable to neutralization by family interaction during the subsequent days. When Mary reentered the family scene on her own that night, she set up a rebirth prototype for that final freedom to establish a new family without living either a lifetime of hate for her parents or of triangular chaos between her spouse-to-be and her parents. The therapist had established a new triangle, so that Mary was not tied to her two parents as individuals, but to the new triangle of parents, Mary and therapist. The therapist thus could push Mary into the family and out of it. The new puberty ceremony could be repeated until it yielded mobility for both Mary and the parents (Zuk, 1969).

Jim was an 18-year-old who had attempted suicide—almost successfully—by carbon monoxide in his closed garage. He was seen three days later with his parents, his older sister and his younger brother in a family conference on the closed inpatient ward. The resident summarized current contacts: the boy had been aloof on the ward, obviously not only very depressed, but also pretty disorganized in his thinking and quite unable to talk about his family relationships or the basis for his suicide attempt.

In the family interview, once dad and mother and two kids had tried to define the characteristic living pattern of the family, the patient was asked, "Who in the family wants you dead?"—"Nobody." —"There must be somebody. Nobody attempts suicide except as a two-person event."—"Maybe my dad. He gets awfully mad at the way I treat mother."—"How about that, dad? You think things would be better around the house if your son was dead?"—The family, of course, was horrified. Father protested but after a bit the older sister said she could understand why I asked the question. She also expressed a feeling that maybe her brother's statement was partly true. *Therapist to Jim*: "Hey, what if you had succeeded? Suppose you had really made it. How long would dad grieve?" He hesitated a moment and then said, "Two weeks."—"How long would mother grieve?"—"Two months."—"How about your brother?"—"Quite a while."—"How about your sister?"—"As long as she lives."—"What kind of a funeral would they give you?"—"I don't know."—"Would it be a fancy casket with lots of flowers and lots of people?"—"I suppose so."—"What would they do with your clothes?"—"I don't know. Maybe they'd give them to my brother."—"What about your girl's picture and the other things of your own?"—"They'd probably burn them all."—"What about your room?"—"I don't know."—"Would you want to be buried in the family plot?"—"I guess so."—"Would your girl friend come to the funeral?"—"Probably not."—"You mean she already has another boy friend?"—"I suppose so."

This kind of investigation into the family dynamics of hostility and the direct deliberate contamination of the intrapsychic fantasy of "they'll be sorry when I'm dead and gone" are techniques of family methodology which certainly would be hard to replicate in individual therapy. The fact that mother and father and siblings are present during the fantasy gives it a quality of reality and probably serves as a pretty good immunization against future suicide episodes. The activation of Jim's perception of father's hostility and the direct presentation of his cynicism about mother and one of the siblings will certainly change the overt, and maybe even the covert, dynamics in future family contacts. The therapist is making direct efforts to pull the son back into the family so that they can all work through the final separation process and he can leave constructively rather than by way of the graveyard.

The middle-class family may ask for help. The lower-class family is usually forced to seek help by society, i.e. the school or the police. Such a family may not be available for insight therapy. The therapist may be able to reverse the motion toward a family dropout problem by direct manipulation of the family dynamic pattern.

Bill, 11, was adored by 9-year-old Mike. Father's indifference to the two of them was only equaled by mother's tearful whining. *Mother*: "Bill has been completely out of my control since he was eight. That was a terrible year. My mother died, you know—she did live with us."—*Therapist*: "Dad, can you control Bill?"—*Father*: "I leave the children to mother. They never bother me."—*Therapist*: "Mother, did you ever wonder if he's winking at the boys and sort of laughing at your suffering?"—*Mother*: "Well, we've had a rough time too. Sometimes he acts like he hates me."—*Therapist*: "Did he hate your mother?"—*Mother*: "Yes, they fought all the time."—*Therapist*: "And now you're the mother so he's fighting a cold war with you through the kids. Maybe if you decided to be the mother you could take over with the kids."—*Bill*: "If she fights us Dad'll slap her face like he did Grandma's."—*Mother*: "Shut up, Bill. Your father has never raised a hand to me and he'd better not either."—*Bill*: "Shut your damned face, maw." Suddenly Father's hand flipped. The back of it bounced off Bill's nose. "I don't like your talking to maw that way." Tears flowed—of relief in mother's eyes—of consternation in Bill's. His moment of terror ended the interview. The flight into health was more gradual but the direction was set.

T.J., 35, decided to send his wife, also 35, to see a psychiatrist. The therapist insisted that he also come for the initial interview. The story of their 13 years of fight training was filled with ghosts of near tragedy and bittersweet yen for revenge. When planning for the second meeting the therapist insisted that they bring the four children. This seemed senseless to the parents but they accepted the mandate. The children were a surprise—gentle, verbal, outgoing and congenial with each other, the parents and the two therapists. The parents opened up the third or report interview by demanding: "So what was the use of having the kids in?" The therapist replied, "That was the clincher in this evaluation. You folks can keep on talking about your pain but never again can you make us wonder if your pain is covering serious pathology." These parents in the initial contact appeared to be adults with serious pathology. Seeing the children made clear that the problem was a family problem. Subsequent three generation conferences clarified the symbiotic quality of the tie between Mrs. T.J. and her parents which had been the undercover basis for their years of horror. Disruption of the adolescent rebellion between mother and grandmother enabled Mr. and Mrs. T.J. to develop a peer relationship that was non-symbiotic.

These 35-year-old adolescents had never broken with the family feud of their parents. Yet, somehow the third generation seemed to have escaped without gross distortion. How could that be? Was the complementary character structure nourishing? Did the desperate dependence of the grandparents keep the parents from traumatizing the children? We can only theorize about what is taking place, but we do recognize the value of working with as much of the family system as can be pulled together into the reorganization process.

USING A PSEUDO-FAMILY

Since the family is not always available, one may be forced to work with a pseudo-family. The peer mates many times offer a friendship network which has many similarities to the family of origin. Just as in marriage, there are both a projected intrapsychic family scene on the part of each person and a defined role.

> Mike was referred by his parents from a distant city. They said he had come home after being sent by his colleagues following an attempt at suicide by carbon monoxide. The author saw the patient and his family for the initial interview. The family then went back a thousand miles to their home with the understanding that Mike would be seen with his "pad." The pad consisted of six boys and one girl; the girl seemed more directly related to Sam although all assumed she was really just one of the group. When it was pointed out that one of the members had attempted suicide and they were partially responsible for this near tragedy, they showed considerable concern and some sense of responsibility. The evidence of their family quality included the fact that they had lived in the same rooms for 2½ years. Sam was the only one who did any cooking. He cooked two meals a week. He turned out to be bitterly angry at the fact that in the whole 2½ years, no one had ever offered to wash the dishes, even once.
>
> It was clear to this group that Mike had drifted away from them and that they had been irritated by his walking through the group and going down to the cellar to play his guitar for four hours. It was equally clear that their bitterness with him was one of the things which precipitated his attempting to take his life. As a matter of fact, they were so angry at him and at each other that they were unwilling to go along with the offer to participate in family therapy. The author's failure to induce them to go on with family therapy made the subsequent individual treatment much less effective, since the dynamics of the group were partly responsible for the stress that precipitated the suicide attempt.

It may be possible to construct a surrogate family from living associates of the identified patient—a ghetto school class or the neighborhood primary interest group makes therapy a social group process. The addition of social workers or recreation workers may help expand the conference to include the disconnected family who will always be crucial to success.

Current psychotherapy of adolescents is frequently based on the concept that the family should be a resource for the adolescent. The therapist's problem then would be to increase the lovingness, increase the availability, increase the denial of self within the family group so that the adolescent can fill his emotional needs before he leaves. I contend that this effort is a mistake. The family members also have a right to their living process; they have a right to group loyalty, as well as individual initiative and liberation. There is no reason why they should be subjugated to the rebellious defiance of the teenager. The family needs the therapist's support to be hostile and to be loving. They must demand the right to be a group and the right to be individuals. This should be the byproduct of a good experience in family therapy. It helps the scapegoat reenter his family of origin, complete his individuation in coordination with other family members, and graduate with honors.

REFERENCES

FLESCHER, J. (1968). Dual analysis. In *Current Psychiatric Therapies*, 8:38-46. Jules H. Masserman, ed. New York: Grune and Stratton.

WHITAKER, C. A., and MILLER, M. H. (1969). A re-evaluation of psychiatric help when divorce impends. *American Journal of Psychiatry*, 126:611-618.

ZUK, GERALD K. (1969). Critical evaluation of triadic-based family therapy. *International Journal of Psychiatry*, 8:539-548, 560-569.

14

Object-Oriented Approaches to Severely Disturbed Adolescents

HYMAN SPOTNITZ, M.D., Med.Sc.D.

Contradictory opinions on the response of adolescents to analytic psychotherapy, and even doubts about their "true analyzability," have been reported. The literature also stresses the paradoxical nature of the differential diagnosis of psychopathology and the transitory emotional upheavals experienced on the developmental level between puberty and adulthood. The rite of passage from late childhood to early maturity is characteristically associated with the use of defenses that are often difficult to differentiate from florid symptoms.

The inherently problematic nature of the transition from childhood to adulthood is suggested in formulations that link symptomatology with normality—for example, Anthony's (1970) reference to the "normal depression of adolescence" or Sugar's (1968) theory of "normal adolescent mourning"—and by Anna Freud's (1958) identification of the absence of turmoil at this stage of life as an indication for treatment. As she has pointed out, "Adolescent manifestations come close to symptom formation of the neurotic, the psychotic or dissocial order and merge almost imperceptibly into borderline states, initial, frustrated or fully fledged forms of almost all the mental illnesses."

Undoubtedly, psychic reactions to the attainment of physical genitality and the reproductive capacity, coupled with the reawakening of pregenital impulses, confront the practitioner with problems he does not

---

This paper is based on a paper and workshop conducted at the Conference of the American Society for Adolescent Psychiatry in New Orleans on January 15, 1971. An earlier version of that paper has appeared in *Progress in Group and Family Therapy*, edited by Clifford Sager, M.D. and Helen Singer Kaplan, M.D., Ph.D., Brunner/Mazel, 1972.

have to contend with in the treatment of children or adults. The process of detachment from parents and experimental approaches to new love objects are reflected in rapid fluctuations in the transference relationship. The adolescent's wish to be helped is typically stronger than that of the child. So too is the mental suffering of the adolescent, and in many cases he mobilizes powerful and subtle defenses against experiencing it.

Another reason why psychotherapy in this critical phase is complex is that the patient is part child, part adult. To treat him as a child is to insult the adult components of his personality; to treat him as an adult entails some degree of failure in meeting the maturational needs of the child. Even though the general principles of psychotherapy with adults are applicable, each adolescent presents a special problem and has to be understood as an individual.

The large number of failures reported in the treatment of adolescents has built up the impression that they are unsuitable candidates for analytic therapy. The major reason for these failures, however, appears to be the tendency to expose these patients to undue pressure for progress. Usually they respond favorably when their vulnerability to the development of high states of tension is borne in mind and they are permitted to proceed at their own pace.

In supervisory work I find that therapists who report difficulties in working with adolescents have usually been trying to get them to *do something*. Typically, the psychotherapist beginning to work with this age group demonstrates, in one way or another, great interest in helping the patient improve his immediate functioning. That attitude often leads to disappointment, because, as the adolescent begins to "unwind," his behavior tends to worsen. When, on the other hand, he gets the message that the therapist is more interested in dealing with obstacles to cooperative communication that the patient encounters in the relationship than in helping him change his behavior, the case proceeds more smoothly. Given permission to be himself, the adolescent eventually becomes interested in understanding what is going on in the relationship; at that point, he begins to make noticeable improvement.

By and large, the approaches that are most effective with teenagers are less stimulating than those employed with children. The therapist needs to maintain an exploratory attitude and use interpretation sparingly. He intervenes only when the patient asks for information or when a communication is clearly required to preserve the relationship.

In operational terms, the main problem in treatment of the adolescent is the failure of the customary interpretive procedures to resolve his resistances to communicating freely. He presents special patterns of resistance that do not respond directly to understanding and insight because they are upheld by powerful maturational needs. At a time when the ego is in a state of rapid flux, explanations of immature functioning are traumatizing and at times have a paralyzing effect. Interpretations mobilize a great deal of aggression, thus stimulating aggressive acting out.

But when these age-specific resistances are dealt with *indirectly*—that is, by facilitating the resolution of the maturational needs that maintain the patterns and by helping the patient verbalize his aggressive impulses —movement in the direction of personality maturation gets under way. The indirect approach may resolve the resistance only temporarily, but it reduces his need to resist. In short, interventions are based on recognition of the patient's resistances and defenses as attempts to control aggression or as the products of maturational needs (Spotnitz, 1969).

That recognition dictates a more time-consuming approach to resistance than exerting analytic pressure on the patient to overcome it; however, the more regressed the patient, the greater his need for the indirect approach when he enters treatment. Eventually he is able to profit from insight and asks for it; interpretations of his defective functioning are then helpful rather than ego-damaging.

Adolescents with mild oedipal-type disturbances are responsive to individual, group, or family treatment. Those with severe psychoneuroses, behavior disorders, character disturbances, schizophrenia, and other preoedipal conditions are not equally responsive to these modes of treatment. Combined treatment is indicated in some of these cases. In order to achieve the degree of specificity required to resolve these problems, careful evaluation of each patient is essential. The therapeutic approaches discussed in this chapter are generally applicable to adolescents with deteriorating conditions.

Individual psychotherapy is indicated for the emotionally overcharged adolescent, who requires little stimulation from the environment. The therapist facilitates the maintenance of a calm treatment climate by timing and formulating his communications to reflect the patient's "contact functioning"—that is, his conscious and unconscious attempts to elicit a response—and by intervening primarily to deal with questions posed by the patient. When contact functioning is employed as a guide to interventions, the patient is, in a sense, provided with emotional feeding on a self-demand schedule. For example, a highly excitable teenager for whom this approach was very reassuring was an obese youth who developed a pattern of overeating to relieve his anxieties. Assisted to talk without interruption in a kind but cool climate, he became less anxious and was able to moderate his food intake.

Obviously it is easier to provide communication on a self-demand basis in the one-to-one relationship than in a group. Some adolescents, however, cannot tolerate a situation in which there is little communication from the therapist. This problem may arise in the individual psychotherapy of an emotionally hungry, narcissistic adolescent with strongly regressive tendencies. Although he may later require individual treatment to deal with his more intimate problems, he is usually more immediately responsive to a group therapeutic experience.

Unlike the schizophrenic adult, who tolerates long periods of silence and minimal communication from the therapist, the schizophrenic adolescent tends to either regress or become explosive in a non-stimulating treatment climate. In the absence of immediate emotional communication, he may activate primitive defenses or his condition may become static. It is easier to provide him with the additional emotional stimulation he needs in the group setting, where other patients confront him with different reactions simultaneously. He can be placed in an adult group, but one composed exclusively of adolescents is preferable when the need for friends—peer reinforcement—is primary.*

Group treatment is also indicated for the drug-prone teenager. Such drugs as marijuana and the amphetamines appear to neutralize the influence of the therapist as transference object. In relatively benign cases, the patient may give up the drug after a series of individual sessions, but serious addictions are more responsive to a group experience with peers who do not take drugs.

In either treatment setting, the severely disturbed adolescent often activates patterns of resistance that are intractable to the customary therapeutic procedures. The pathologically narcissistic patient becomes preoccupied with his defective ego functioning and tends to control his aggression by withdrawing psychologically from the treatment situation (Spotnitz, 1969). A special approach to this resistance is often required to counter his introspective tendencies.

OBJECT-ORIENTED QUESTIONING

Retrospectively I recognize that the orientation discussed here was suggested by my early experience with patients beginning treatment in a psy-

---

* Therapeutic management in adolescent group therapy is the subject of an excellent report by Leslie Rosenthal (1971).

chotic state. They were usually incapable of talking, let alone talking about themselves in an emotionally meaningful way. Given some assistance, however, they were able to talk about inconsequential subjects, and this proved to be a relatively efficient way of establishing contact with them. They were therefore asked many questions about numerous aspects of their daily routine—for example, what they had eaten for breakfast, how they had slept, whether hospital attendants or family members were giving them proper care, and the like. As long as the labile phase lasted, they were asked only about aspects of their current activities that would have been perceived by an ever-present and observant companion. Such questioning helped to bring them out of psychosis relatively quickly, and also proved effective in the early stage of treatment when they tended to relapse.

In working with patients in post-psychotic conditions, it is sometimes necessary to help them talk first about external events and other impersonal matters. For example, a man who had expressed eagerness to address himself to his emotional problems during the initial interview, and was otherwise able to comply with the requirements for office treatment, was unable to express himself coherently during his first year of psychotherapy. Although the last of several courses of electroshock therapy he had undergone had been completed some years earlier, he still betrayed their mentally disorganizing effects. When he was too troubled or confused by his jumbled ideas to answer questions, I talked to him about external realities such as current events, books, and the theater. After the psychic obstacles to the formation of a cooperative treatment relationship were thus gradually resolved, he was able to apply himself effectively to his emotional problems.

Object-oriented investigations have special values for the severely disturbed adolescent, particularly one in late adolescence. He is hypersensitive to direct probing into his problems. If one tries to induce him to talk about them, he often feels that he is being put "on the spot." He then becomes more anxious and feels more resentful about whatever is bothering him at the moment. On the other hand, interventions that do not focus on his deficiencies and difficulties are very reassuring to him. Moreover, when his attention is repeatedly directed to other persons or emotionally insignificant aspects of his daily experience, he becomes curious about why his problems are not being investigated. One adolescent said, "I don't see how it's going to help me to talk about football and the war in Vietnam." Another patient became annoyed after being questioned at length about a schoolmate he had met at the movies that week. He asked, "Why should I waste time telling you his name and what he looks like? Why don't we talk about the things that are troubling me?" That was the first time resentful feelings were verbalized by these patients, and the first time they demonstrated the ability to communicate freely.

Group treatment is by its very nature an object-oriented experience. Each participant has just a fraction of the time to talk about himself and drifts naturally in the direction of involvement with his co-patients. Since group processes militate against prolonged self-preoccupation, the group therapist is not called on to do much talking to check it. In those relatively rare situations when an intervention is indicated for that purpose, however, there are various ways he may intervene to draw the patient's attention to his present objects. The therapist may, for example, ask someone else a question or "go around" the group inviting each of its members to verbalize his impressions of another person's functioning or problems. Consequently, it is more difficult for a patient to remain self-absorbed and uncommunicative in the group.

From time to time, one encounters an adolescent who is totally unresponsive to treatment. Neither individual nor group therapy checks his deterioration, and he continues to indulge in behavior that is dangerous to himself or others. In such a case, it may be necessary to investigate the responsiveness of that patient to an experimental procedure.

CONSTRUCTIVE EMOTIONAL INTERCHANGE

One such procedure, evolving from the object-oriented approach, is conceptualized as constructive emotional interchange. Although its application is not limited to adolescents, their age-specific vulnerability to self-disclosure and defensively hostile attitudes to adults make them ideal candidates for the procedure. It has been effectively employed with several adolescents, and its application is discussed here in the context of that age group.

Constructive emotional interchange emancipates the adolescent from the role of patient. The implementation of this operational principle is highly specific, depending on the adolescent's underlying problem, current reality situation, and reactions to the other participants in the interchanges—usually both parents and, when appropriate, his siblings. But regardless of the overt content of these verbal exchanges, the adolescent is not asked to talk about himself and attention is directed away from his intrapsychic problems. He is helped, instead, to deal with the problems he creates for the family. The therapist structures the sessions to bring into strong focus the reactions of the participating family members to the adolescent's behavior and to help him deal with these reactions.

Despite the participation of family members in constructive emotional interchange, I do not regard it as a variant of family therapy. "In its strictest sense," Ackerman (1972) stated, "the term family therapy refers to a systematic method of psychotherapeutic intervention, designed to alleviate the multiple, interlocking emotional disorders of a family group." Constructive emotional interchange is based on a principle that can be broadly applied in both family and group psychotherapy, but the specific application discussed here is not family therapy in the sense of the strict definition just mentioned. The family members who participate are not diagnosed; their problems are not investigated or discussed, except tangentially and in terms of their effect on the adolescent. The presence of family members is essentially a therapeutic tool for treating the adolescent indirectly, that is, in terms of their current reactions to his behavior. Constructive emotional interchange is therefore viewed as treatment of the young patient in the family setting.

Even if one equates the use of the family setting with family therapy,* it is questionable strategy to refer to the procedure discussed here as such when one tries to secure the participation of the adolescent's family in constructive emotional interchange. In some instances, the parents cooperate only because they think their presence will eventually be helpful to the patient; they are motivated solely by their anxieties about his condition, anxieties that effectively mask whatever problems they may have. They do not regard themselves as candidates for psychotherapy and they do not want it; the notion that the family is to be dealt with as a treatment unit would give rise to insurmountable resistances in these parents. On the other hand, the formulation that constructive emotional interchange would help another member of the family evokes a favorable response in the parent, as in the adolescent.

Constructive emotional interchange with the adolescent is predicated on two observations:

---

* Where family therapy begins and where it ends has yet to be determined. It is still, in Ackerman's words (1972), an "extremely fuzzy" field. In one of his later communications on the subject, which includes the strict definition of family therapy quoted above, he more loosely identifies as family therapy ten diverse psychotherapeutic procedures that entail the participation of the family. Constructive emotional interchange could be covered under a few of these broader definitions.

1. Whereas the dominant problem of the adult patient relates in some way to his adjustment to society, that of the adolescent is contending with his inner urges. At this stage of life, the magnification of feelings, especially those that he does not want to experience, may cause excruciating suffering. The task of dealing with his endogenous impulses is compounded when he is bombarded with feelings of people around him that he cannot assimilate healthfully. A refusal to experience these feelings may drive him into deviant forms of behavior. And the tendency of the adolescent to act on feelings is exacerbated by the new dangers that beset mankind today—the technological threats to human survival, as well as the new sexual freedom, the overstimulating effects of information on violent acts, and the greater availability of drugs, knives, and guns.

2. Parents are highly significant objects to the adolescent. For many years I have been impressed with the need demonstrated by young people recovering from severe emotional disturbance to influence their parents, help them release feelings, and change them. After verbalizing such wishes, they often add, "if only I knew how!" The need to reach out and help a parent is strong in the adolescent who was exposed to a great deal of positive feeling, which was so inconsistently or inappropriately communicated that the desire to reciprocate it was stifled.

In constructive emotional interchange, the customary policy of enlisting the cooperation of parents on behalf of the patient is reversed. The young patient is cast in the role of helper. The therapist so manages the interviews that the adolescent takes the initiative in helping his parents deal with their feelings. He assists them in verbalizing their feelings for him with awareness and regard for his reactions to their communications.

This procedure is tailored to provide the emotional ingredients needed by the emotionally hungry adolescent with narcissistic problems. The greater his desire to help his parents—whether or not he is conscious of this desire—the more responsive he is to the procedure. The parents who qualify for constructive emotional interchange are those who have appropriate feelings for the patient and can be educated to control their expression. Usually they have exposed him to feelings at the wrong time or in the wrong dosage, or they may have lacked the verbal facility to communicate these feelings effectively. The participants may also include siblings of the patient, provided that they too demonstrate strong interest in committing themselves to mutually helpful communication.

The parents must eventually agree not to verbally assault or to humiliate the patient in the sessions. Untimely or overly strong expressions of feelings may overwhelm the adolescent and may stimulate suicidal impulses in him, as well as rebelliousness, accidents, and behavior destructive to others.

The treatment is structured to provide a non-damaging and mutually beneficial experience. The value for the parents is that, in the process of being trained to provide the kind of psychological food the patient needs at the tempo he can digest it, they secure his help in controlling their communications. The patient benefits in four ways: (1) functioning in the role of helper boosts his ego; (2) the feelings he helps his parents verbalize appropriately serve to meet his maturational needs; (3) in working on their problems, he discovers problems of his own that he would not otherwise be willing to recognize as such, and is thus able to accept help for himself; and (4) the feelings of love that are communicated to him by the parents serve to greatly increase his self-esteem.

The clinical material that follows illustrates the use of this object-oriented, investigative procedure in the treatment of an adolescent who had not benefited from individual psychotherapy or hospitalization.

CLINICAL ILLUSTRATION

A bright, somewhat moody boy, Paul had been a model student and seemed to be developing favorably until the age of twelve. The emergence of his emotional problems coincided with the departure of his older sister from home. He then became the focus of his parents' attention, at times receiving more of it than he wanted and at other times being neglected because of their active social life. Both individually and as a team, they handled him inconsistently.

His mother, an attractive and energetic woman, was inclined to act on impulse. When her impetuous behavior got her into difficulties, she would become frightened and try to reverse herself. Paul reacted to her occasional attempts to discipline him by locking himself in his room or storming out of the house. The father, a successful manufacturer, was given to fits of anger. He oscillated between entrusting Paul's mother with full responsibility for his upbringing and suddenly stripping her of that responsibility when Paul defied her. Though the parents were happy together in many respects, their son's behavior had become a source of much friction between them.

Paul began individual psychotherapy at the age of twelve, when his emotional problems became apparent, but he continued to deteriorate. Although he expressed willingness to cooperate at the start, he soon manifested strong resistances to communicating, withholding important information from the psychiatrist. The individual treatment was terminated when the patient attempted suicide—a panic reaction to threats from boys with whom he was taking drugs. He was 14 years old at that time.

Paul was hospitalized after the suicide attempt, the culmination of a series of failures at school and growing strife at home. He had been truanting from school to go on drug trips with cronies whom his parents regarded as undesirable companions, and was taking money from his father's wallet to pay for pep pills and pot. When reprimanded for his failing grades, Paul threatened to drop out of school. Although he was a talented violinist, he had already dropped his music studies. But hospitalization also failed to check his deterioration. Within a year he was transferred from one hospital to another and discharged from the second, after several months, as an incurable schizophrenic.

At this juncture, his parents, greatly alarmed, again consulted the psychiatrist. A series of family interviews was proposed, with the idea that the son would take a leading role in investigating and helping his parents deal with their anxieties about him. Confronted with the alternative of a third hospitalization—this time in a state mental institution—Paul expressed willingness to cooperate to that extent, though he had no confidence that the interviews would be of any help to him.

During these sessions, conducted weekly, rules of conduct that were calculated to allay parental alarm were enunciated as needed. Each deviation from the rules was studied and, when the reason for it was understood, attempts were made to correct it. For example, the parents agreed to restrain their expressions of anger since these tended to heighten the general state of alarm. When the father exploded in rage, Paul told him to "cool it" and explored with him the reason for the outburst. Over a period of months, it was discovered that the father's explosive anger was connected with fears provoked by Paul's frequent misunderstanding of his directions, and by the mother's evident anxieties. Another rule, occasionally implemented to help the mother control her impulsivity, was that she was not to talk until Paul gave her permission to do so. His feeling of being stifled by her gradually diminished, and he developed a sense of power and control in their relations.

One of the major sources of disturbance in the family was each member's misperception of the feelings of the others. Paul, for instance, interpreted his mother's nagging at him to stop smoking pot as an attempt on her part to impose her will and deprive him of freedom of action; he did not recognize that she was reacting to intense fears that he was damaging himself. Similarly, his father's anxieties and explosions of anger induced feelings in Paul that his father was trying to humiliate him, and he characteristically reacted to these feelings by avoiding contact with his father. Initially the youth insisted that, if his parents had the right to drink Scotch, he was entitled to take drugs. The parents viewed this attitude as a deliberate defiance of their wishes, whereas the son saw himself as being merely self-assertive. Their strong pressure for compliance, he said, obliged him to make an effort to assert himself. Furthermore, he contended that he had a right to do anything that would make life more tolerable for him. In view of his manifest difficulties, their highly emotional reactions irritated him and he considered them to be inappropriate.

In the sessions, Paul demonstrated growing interest in helping his mother resolve her tendency to behave impulsively when frightened. He became more and more aware of the connection between his own behavior and her acute anxiety; eventually, he realized that she nagged him because she was anxious. He verbalized feelings of sympathy for her plight and then, after the interviews had been conducted for several months, moved forward from sympathy to action. He announced that he would give up drugs in order to relieve her. He said he did not really need drugs.

This dramatic change of attitude greatly reassured his mother and transformed the emotional climate of the home. Equally notable were the steady improvement in Paul's performance at school and his more discriminating choice of companions. He formed new friendships with boys his parents approved of. Before the end of the first year of interviews, he had resumed his music lessons and was contemplating a career as a violinist under the aegis of an outstanding teacher.

Discussion

To review the psychodynamic factors underlying the sequence of events just described:

When Paul agreed to help his parents deal with their feelings, he did not believe the psychiatrist's statement that helping them in this way might help him too. Nothing else had worked for him, so the "crazy" psychiatrist had dreamed up that scheme. But he agreed to participate to avoid being rehospitalized.

When the interchanges with his parents heated up, he began to study the effects of their feelings on him and his feelings on them. It slowly became clear to him that what he had personally experienced as verbal attacks were, from their point of view, the involuntary responses of concerned parents who really loved him and had trouble dealing with the fears he stirred up in them by getting himself into precarious situations. Increasing recognition of their affection and concern stimulated strong desires in Paul to allay their anxieties.

Later he came to recognize that these anxieties were also affecting his parents' behavior toward him outside the interviews and accounted for many of the restraints they imposed on him. It dawned on Paul that his difficulties in getting along with them waxed and waned somewhat with their emotional states. He experienced them as reasonable, even benevolent, when they were relatively free from anxiety, whereas he felt that he was being crushed by iron hands when they were wrought up about his behavior, as they frequently were.

Paul also discovered that their anxieties about him were adversely affecting their own relationship. They spoke despairingly at times of having failed with him. Occasionally one parent blamed the other for Paul's problems. His mother verbalized feelings of worthlessness that induced intense rage in his father. In the course of investigating the emotional influence that each parent was exerting on the other and on himself, Paul experienced wishes to relieve their suffering and to disengage himself from patterns of behavior that were triggering conflict between them. These wishes grew stronger as the interviews continued.

After he understood the marital stress in which he was a factor and became aware of his power to alleviate it, Paul wanted to help his parents deal with emotional difficulties in which he was not directly implicated. He became interested in knowing them as people—not just as parents. He questioned his father about business matters, his mother about community causes to which she devoted much time. Their openness to his opinions and suggestions regarding their pursuits, especially their responsiveness in terms of behavior, made it seem more natural to him that they should guide him in managing his own life.

As Paul began to feel more at ease about venturing into areas of his parents' lives beyond the home with suggestions for changes, his rebellious defiance gave way to cooperative self-assertiveness. His ability to help his parents master the expression of their feelings and to allay their anxieties gave him some confidence that he could play a favorable role in their lives. The parents, by meeting Paul's maturational need for expressions of warm positive feelings—love, admiration, and respect—made it easier for him to improve his behavior.

Any new experience has the potential for reorganizing existing memories. New and ego-syntonic emotional interchanges with parents during the labile period of adolescence may thus reduce the tension connected with the developmental task of separation-individuation. Sugar (1968), focusing on one aspect of that task, has theorized that depressive moods and various other affective manifestations reflect those processes by which the adolescent mourns for "the parents from whom he is separating—the lost infantile objects." Adaptation to that loss appears to be facilitated for the adolescent who, in the process of giving up his infantile objects, gains objects that are both similar and dissimilar—like the lost objects in that they are his real parents, and different in that they now function to meet his present maturational needs.

Mourning reactions did not figure prominently in the case of Paul; they were overshadowed by his strivings to rid himself of the influence of the old objects. But he was glad to accept his parents' influence as new and different objects. Given the opportunity to explore their current reactions to him, the youth acquired impressions that were more favorable than his past impressions of them. The new impressions were a powerful therapeutic force.

The remarkable improvement observed in Paul's functioning at the end of the first year of constructive emotional interchange greatly surprised him. He did not concede that this could have resulted from the change in his parents' behavior. After two years of constructive emotional interchange, it was easier for him to recognize that mutual helpfulness and understanding can produce significant alterations in all of the participants. During the third year, a subject that has frequently come up for discussion is the mother's inability to lose weight, as recommended by her physician. After she had volunteered information about her lack of progress, Paul helped her select a diet that she would be most likely to adhere to and then helped her to do so. In a situation when she was reporting progress, he interrupted her to direct attention to a problem he was becoming aware of in his social life. He reported various difficulties in forming good relationships with girls, and added, "Do you know, I really think now that I need some treatment myself."

But this statement reflected an attempt to escape from the family situation rather than a strong desire to accelerate his improvement. It is possible that Paul, now nearing his twenties, will develop a firm resolve to work on his fundamental problem in individual analytic psychotherapy. At the present time, however, he continues to meet with his parents.

CONCLUDING OBSERVATIONS

Constructive emotional interchange emerges as a byproduct of controlling communication in the interviews in terms of its effects on the patient. Interventions are made primarily to influence the timing and dosage of expressions of feelings by members of the adolescent's family, so that the emotional ingredients that he wants and needs are verbalized in ways that make him feel more secure.

The therapist operates on the assumption that the adolescent who experiences certain types of communications from his parents as agreeable and other types as disagreeable will strive to alter the conditions that lead to the disagreeable emotional reactions. The adolescent does not see his own behavior as a problem; what he does recognize as the problem is his parents' behavior. He would like them to experience feelings that would enable them to relate to him in a consistently agreeable manner. In the sessions he becomes aware of their positive feelings for him and his own positive feelings for them. These feelings stimulate him to change his behavior.

Exchanges of positive feelings, combined with assistance in verbalizing them, help the adolescent deal with his conflicts in ways that make inner change possible. The process of learning to communicate with his parents in mutually agreeable ways becomes so rewarding, personally and socially, that he develops strong desires to preserve these gains. When constructive emotional interchange with highly significant objects becomes ego-syntonic, the patient really wants to work to resolve his own emotional problems.

The adolescent's willingness to help his parents deal with their feelings, and their reciprocal need to help him and cooperate with him in his efforts to help them are the fundamental prerequisites for this approach. The existence of these attitudes opens up the possibility of resolving one of the major obstacles to harmonious family relations—that is, the inability of family members to influence each other's feelings agreeably. Addressing itself consistently to this problem, constructive emotional interchange equips the therapist with a powerful instrument for improving the adolescent's functioning in the family milieu and also in his social relationships.

REFERENCES

ACKERMAN, N. W. (1972). The growing edge of family therapy. In *Progress in Group and Family Therapy*, C. J. Sager and H. S. Kaplan, eds., pp. 440-456. New York: Brunner/Mazel.

ANTHONY, E. J. (1970). Two contrasting types of adolescent depressions and their treatment. *Journal of the American Psychoanalytic Association,* 18:841-859.

FREUD, A. (1958). Adolescence. *Psychoanalytic Study of the Child,* 13:225-278.

ROSENTHAL, L. (1971). Some dynamics of resistance and therapeutic management in adolescent group therapy. *Psychoanalytic Review,* 58:353-366.

SPOTNITZ, H. (1969). *Modern Psychoanalysis of the Schizophrenic Patient.* New York: Grune and Stratton.

SPOTNITZ, H. (1972). Constructive emotional interchange in adolescence. In *Progress in Group and Family Therapy,* C. J. Sager and H. S. Kaplan, eds., pp. 737-746. New York: Brunner/Mazel.

SUGAR, M. (1968). Normal adolescent mourning. *American Journal of Psychotherapy,* 22:258-269.

15

Combined Family and Group Therapy for Problems of Adolescents: A Synergistic Approach

DAVID MENDELL, M.D.

Among the continual challenges in the field of psychotherapy are the questions of how to develop new techniques, find effective combinations of them, and evaluate these methods of treatment. From the various modalities that have developed in the recent history of psychotherapy at least three distinct patterns seem to have emerged: (1) traditional individual therapy; (2) family therapy; and (3) group psychotherapy. The concept which I wish to submit for consideration is a combination of family and group therapy for the disturbed adolescent. This synergistic approach[*] integrates and converges several systems rather than any one and includes the personal system of the therapist as extensively as possible.

This alternative, in my personal clinic experience, shows certain promising possibilities. Because the complexities are vast, I shall here touch only on some primary facets.

Perhaps one of the most interesting aspects of Freud's work was the association of success in therapy of a given patient with the strength of his ego. Throughout the history of psychotherapy there has always been the question of whether persons with egos of limited strength could successfully complete psychotherapy. Thus, a number of psychotherapists have restricted eligibility of such patients to supportive rather than indepth therapy. Those of us interested in group therapy and family therapy

---

[*] R. Buckminster Fuller defines synergy as behavior of whole systems unpredicted by the behavior of any or several of the system's parts. For me it is that the combination is more than the sum of the parts taken alone (see also Mendell, 1973).

231

also recognize that the patient with a reasonably intact ego who returns after his therapeutic sessions to a sufficiently disruptive family situation may not be able to function satisfactorily, whereas if the patient were completely autonomous, the chances of successful therapy would be much greater. To Freud's original concern about the relative degree of ego strength, we add the degree of family integration. Elsewhere (Fisher and Mendell, 1956; Mendell and Fisher, 1956) I have developed this concept in some detail, showing transgenerationally how the families may be integrative or disintegrative as a result of a historical transmission of affective patterns. The family structure must be considered as a crucial factor in the course of therapy.

Theoretically, the synergistic approach can be represented by the concept of "sharing the burden" of the therapeutic process, a corrective and integrative modality reestablished as a goal for the individual, as well as the family (group) or organization, and carried through into the contiguous or successive relationships, such as outside groups or succeeding generations. If the stress and burden of therapy could be shared by all members of a family of a patient seeking therapy—even though some may not have a very intact ego, or even though the family structure may be relatively disintegrated—then we may not only help resolve the problems of the patient, but also help convert a disintegrated family structure into an integrated one.

INDICATIONS AND CONSIDERATIONS

Whereas this approach should work with anyone involved in the psychotherapeutic process, the following are the situations in which it would be most commonly indicated.

Because of his dependency the child is not equipped to carry the burden of therapy alone. The troubled adolescent has still not solved his relationship to his family nor his separation from it. His parents, on the other hand, may be threatened by his change or growth.

Secondly, certain psychotics clearly represent patients with Freud's "incomplete ego." Here, again, we have a child in the psychotic man, who, therefore, needs more "sharing of the burden."

Thirdly, the decompensated adult—also with an incomplete ego—requires similar support.

Finally, patients should be included who, regardless of the strength of ego, live in a family situation that is sufficiently disintegrated or disruptive to impair seriously the progress of conventional therapy.

With this broad theoretical rationale for the system and classification of the kinds of patients who can benefit the most from combined treatment, I should like to describe this technique as it has developed in my practice through more than 25 years of therapeutic experience with more than 1,000 families. My own clinical experience, related in fairly subjective terms, must certainly be separated from the empirical scientific observations needed for their validation.

The following discussion should distinguish between the approach recommended here and the sole use of family or any other therapy. The more tools the therapist has available, the more situations he can handle effectively. To be bound to any one modality is obviously limiting. The therapist should therefore determine:

1) Which modalities he handles well, from the standpoint of personal aptitude and preference, as well as adequacy of experience with it;

2) To which situations and at what times he will apply the various modalities.

The personal system of the therapist needs to be matched with the presenting patient system. This would appear to be a logical starting point for evaluation of a method of therapy. For example, a therapist who was a youngest brother habitually looking to older siblings for leadership may have difficulty leading a therapy group, and may therefore be unable to evaluate this modality for a given patient with objectivity. Or a novice practitioner who has recently arranged one therapy group will not be as able to prescribe this therapy as a more experienced therapist who has a variety of groups and schedules available. In 1949, when I conducted my first group at the San Francisco Veterans Administration, the primary criterion was that the veteran be available on Monday mornings at 9:30, since this was my consultation morning there.

After experience of the therapist and availability of his group are considered, there is the matter of timing. As in a bridge game, experience is required to go from one modality to another to use available opportunities. First, a constructive relationship with the therapist must be provided for the adolescent and the significant family members. Then, only when appropriate therapy group situations are available, and the therapist feels the family member can benefit from it, should group therapy be undertaken. With reasonable practice he will know when and how to accomplish this step. He may even offer participation in more than one therapy group (Berger and Mendell, 1967).

The next task for the therapist is to achieve a common goal with the "patient" and the rest of the family. This means modifying the request of "treating a patient" to changing the way the family operates. It is important not to overstress the tolerance of the family, lest they take flight. Clarification of the long-term goals will usually motivate the family to stick with the therapy long enough to accomplish what is necessary.

The parents are requested to come in with the adolescent patient. The reply, however, may be negative: the father is out of town, angry, or does not want to have anything to do with the therapy. If the caller, then, is the mother, she is asked to come in with the young patient. And if she says he will not come in either, then she is asked to come in herself. The caller is usually the most anxious family member and the one most motivated for change. Usually, once the initiator is encouraged and reinforced, the rest of the family will come, after one or several sessions. In my view, any help in regard to the problem area for any family member is a means for channeling help to the entire family (Fisher and Mendell, 1958).

THE PSYCHIATRIC FAMILY EVALUATION

This procedure is explained to whoever comes to the first session. Since a family is a team, whatever any one member manifests will somehow be related to the whole team. In a basketball game, for example, if the forward fails to score in his usual way, we would take a look at the rest of the team, as well as the forward. Perhaps the guard is not passing the ball; perhaps there is some dissension in the team; the coach may be troubled and irritated with the team.

The evaluation consists of the observation and study of the family system as a whole and the individual subsystems within it, that is, the subgroupings. In one rare instance, for example, the father and mother of the patient were not able to say anything negative or disagreeable about each other, but seemed to be totally in agreement. Their son, at age 13, had gotten drunk for the first time; a year and a half later he had left home in their car; later he stole a truck and demolished it; and at 16 he had gone berserk in an argument with the father and had smashed the car window. He resented the closeness of his perfectionistic parents and felt a need to strike back at them. This is rather unusual, since, generally, there is at least some conflict between the parents of a troubled adolescent. In this instance, the closeness and interdependence of the parents were so great as to exclude the adolescent, and it was this exclusion to which he was reacting.

Seeing the adolescent and each parent separately, as well as the whole family together, initiates the flow of information and conveys to each that he is of interest as an individual in his own right. To insure cooperation, especially of the more resistant member, the therapist must make each person feel that his position in the matter is understood. Whatever subgroupings will yield significant information can be pursued as well.

An experienced psychologist who has worked with me for many years in the family approach does basic projective studies. He relates the studies of each person to the family and to each member, and particularly seeks common themes to define problem areas which they all share. This is a useful means for convincing even recalcitrant family members that they are involved with and share the same problem as the patient. At various points along the line, the therapist ties in apparently random data and feedback as significant information. Much of this can be done before the initial evaluation has been completed.

This technique also shows points of commonality, as, for example, the father who found that he really had the same problem with his father that his son was having with him. Seeing it from an opposite viewpoint, which he had not previously been able to do, increased his awareness of his own involvement and of his sharing of the problem with the boy, so that it became ego-syntonic instead of a foreign body. Then the data from the sessions and the projective studies are integrated and shared with all members present. Relevant aspects of family operations and functions are explained, so as to increase the involvement of each family member, and to relieve feelings of guilt which might stiffen resistance of any individual involved in the mutual effort.

FAMILY DYNAMICS, RELATED TO PROBLEM AND THERAPY

The family may be compared to an organization or production line in which the raw material, a baby, is developed into a finished product, that is, an adequate adult, mate, parent, and social being. To be human is to be imperfect, and every family has its weaknesses, which, when they become operative, may cause difficulty or failure. The weakness can be explained by the lack of a parental model. What the parents did not experience or learn from their family is difficult for them to achieve; the same holds for the parents' parents who also lacked the parental model, and so on through the generations. Furthermore, if parents cannot handle the weakness in an effective way with their adolescent, they offer him no model; he will not be able to handle it with his children; nor will their children, and so on. Hilde Bruch (1973) has demonstrated in 30 years of experience with weight problems that none of her patients who received treatment had a fat child. This is an opportunity, then, for them not only to help themselves with their current problem, but also to avoid possible suffering in the generations to come.

Depending upon the degree of resistance offered and the needs of a particular family, I also share with my patients my observations of the commonality of family problems on the basis of choice of marital partners. This further focuses on the flow or continuity of the family. It is my impression that one seeks a mate with whom one feels at home, who is like home, but better. If this choice entails a commonality of problem it is more than likely that there is a willingness or capacity in the mate to change or accommodate, as opposed to the original family's rigidity, which cannot be altered by the child. The new family, then, continues the work with new resources and hope.

Most people therefore unconsciously tend to marry someone with a common problem who has alternate means or defenses for alleviating or dealing with it. Initially, so long as one or the other marital partner has a way of dealing with or compensating for the mutual problem, that partner can adjust or cover for the other one. But as time goes on, and the relationship deepens, these mechanisms have all been put into use, and there may remain a residue of problems for which neither family of origin has any solutions. The problem may persist, to the frustration and annoyance of both marital partners, who see the source in the other one only. Since the source is in the unconscious, neither partner sees it in himself. The anger and drive for resolution become directed at the mate, with escalating anger and frustration, and are then redirected by each to others around them; children, being available and vulnerable, are the first targets. The adolescent, with his own emergent individuality and the conflicts attendant thereto, becomes a particular target.

I explain to each person the need to attend to his own contribution to the problem, instead of blaming or projecting, which only produces resistance and worsens the situation. At the point where therapy is sought, each mate has exhausted all his own family resources. This is the unique opportunity for each to identify and resolve the problems arising from his own family of origin and to compensate for some of its deficiencies. The therapy group, then, provides increased leverage as a "surrogate family laboratory," in which the added experience of many other families can be channeled and made available to each parent.

The realization that the specific family problems are not insoluble and a better understanding of family function in general create a more hope-ful aura. A rise in spirits and a beginning improvement can often be noted in the adolescent, who has the feeling that his parents are working with him as a team. To a degree he has been unburdened of the problem of the whole family; the parents, having been relieved of guilt, are happier and do not bear down on him as much. Anxieties may persist, however, or be replaced by overoptimism or wishful thinking. The parents may not wish to face up to the necessary changes and work to be done. The follow-up treatment is therefore very important. Some may return at a later date.

> In Dale's case, the parents did not pursue the therapy when she was 14, but returned when she attempted suicide at 19. The father, who had earlier refused to come in, later attended individual and family sessions. The mother, in addition, went into a therapy group earn-estly, continuing after the daughter left her group. Ultimately, she was able to stand up against her husband's transgressions. This en-couraged the girl, who had been very upset and hostile because of her mother's passivity. Only when the mother was completely inde-pendent, could tell the father off about whatever she did not like, and could control her own life, did she leave the group. By this time the daughter, who had been helplessly involved in a love affair, could stand up to her very disturbed fiancé and not allow him to tyran-nize her. She was able to tolerate his leaving her without becoming suicidal when he refused to change his attitude toward her.

FUNCTION OF THE THERAPY GROUP

Initially I put each parent in a separate therapy group, and often delay putting the adolescent in a group until the parents have become firmly rooted in their own groups. There is a tendency for them to regress to their original wishful thinking that the adolescent can solve their com-mon problem for them once he is settled and working in his group. Who-ever drops out may then become the focus of resistance in further therapy.

If there is any lack of enthusiasm or motivation, as there may be, especially in the more intellectualized or compulsive types, I explain the rationale of the therapy group. Each family has its strengths and its weaknesses. The weaknesses, as well as other behavioral patterns, are established early in life, and are relegated to the unconscious. The meanings of "conscious" and "unconscious" often need explanation. Although the unconscious is by far the most prevalent, it is unavailable informationally for necessary change. As in a dark room containing a hassock, light is needed to move or walk around the hassock and thus keep one from stumbling over it repeatedly. These unresolved conflict areas, being in the unconscious, are not accessible at will. The emergence of related material from other and older members of the group who may be well into a given problem causes reverberations in the new members' unconscious, often referred to as "ringing a bell." Other family representatives in the group are stimulated to express relevant material, which further facilitates identification and recall, until a conflict comes into focus.

Being able to focus on and grasp a problem does not enable one to pluck it out or get rid of it, thereby leaving a vacuum. But now a better solution can be sought, by becoming familiar with the backgrounds and patterns of the other group members. In one's own family, the problem may lie in area A, whereas areas B and C may be strong. Joe, another group member, may have no problem in area A; his family problem may be in area B. Or Suzy, whose family problem is in area C, may handle area A very well. And so one tries Joe's and Suzy's ways in the group, at home, at work, on various occasions. If Joe's way works in handling the problem, that way continues to be used, until it is incorporated and becomes a part of one's approach. The old way, then, atrophies with disuse and falls away. Now, as an adult, one can choose which approach is desirable, rather than continue an old pattern that has been passed on from generation to generation, but is now counterproductive.

The patients are told that it takes a half dozen sessions to get the feeling of the group and become acquainted with the members and their problems. They can ask for an individual or family session any time it is needed or desired, or I can call for one. After half a dozen sessions, they usually prefer the group because they feel they get more out of it. But, throughout, the therapy is related to the family and periodically I expect to have sessions with them together or individually. Data from these sessions are later shared with the rest of the group. It is emphasized that cliques, confidences, or pairing outside the group deprive the group of needed information and hinder its primary purpose. Everything significant, including the post-sessions, therefore must be brought back to the group. Conversely, information from the group is channeled into the family.

INTEGRATION OF FAMILY AND GROUP THERAPIES: CASE ILLUSTRATIONS

Don, a 15-year-old boy, was brought in complaining of severe headaches and drowsiness. Increasingly, he was having problems with friends at school and difficulties relating to other people. He refused to return to school after Christmas vacation. He had formerly played with an orchestra and had worked very hard, but when he began to feel pressed by various teachers he started to withdraw. He had been seen shortly before by a child psychologist, who had initially been encouraged by his marginally favorable response, only to find that the boy became rapidly noncommunicative during later sessions until he refused to participate altogether. Projective studies by another psychologist indicated superior intelligence but severe emotional disturbance and schizophrenic thought disorder, attributed to feelings of being undermined by his parents. Individual psychotherapy was strongly recommended to prevent the boy from becoming more severely emotionally disturbed. When this treatment bogged down, the parents sought help from me.

The boy agreed to come in only on the father's promise to give him a stereophonic set. He spoke very little, indicated the questions he was to be asked, and, with an expressionless face, refused to answer others. The mother, who was distressed and pessimistic, feared that the boy had an incurable psychosis. The father, on the other hand, adopted a more positive attitude: "I feel we should get close to him, help him, and understand ourselves." The parents' relationship appeared to be warm and cordial.

In their tests at this time, the parents revealed difficulties that confronted them; each seemed to set up a screen behind which troublesome issues were hidden. For example, the father described the first Rorschach card as a "screen with something behind it; a blind that has something behind it, but I do not know what it is." The mother described one card as "a figure behind a screen, hidden." Some of the mother's hidden features included rebellious and resentful feelings, fantasies of escape from responsibilities, burdens. In addition, there seemed to be uncertainties or confusion about the parental roles, especially about who was the dominant and assertive figure. They were each put in separate groups.

The boy came for the family interview and one individual session. At the psychologist's office, he pretended to be asleep in the waiting room, later came in, but refused to look at the examiner or make any spontaneous response. Six weeks after his parents had begun therapy, he returned for the tests. He made a few descriptive comments and tended to become angry when pushed for a story. The psychologist noted "his easy toleration for incompatible images without concern about their appropriateness. . . ." Fragmentation of his ego structure was exemplified by one of his Rorschach responses: "Two humans or apes, more like shadows, not solid people, or like negatives of a photograph, with parts not clear in the negative, only half a person, not a whole one." The diagnosis of schizophrenia, with a splintered sense of being and self-image, was made at that time.

The patient came in only two times during the third month of the parents' therapy. The problems of the parents with the boy, their individual selves, and each other were the principal topics dealt with.

The father discontinued his group after five months, when he felt he was making good headway with the boy. The mother continued for about another year. Thereafter the son was seen individually for five months at weekly or biweekly intervals. He then consented to join an adolescent group, in which he remained for about three months. Here his need for and fear of girls was plainly manifest. He was extremely sensitive about being laughed at. Deep personality disturbance was still in evidence. However, he was better adjusted and was functioning. Slow but gradual progress for the boy was reported initially, during which time he did not go to school. He kept himself occupied reading intensively, playing his music, and working in his father's business. In the last sessions he smiled and laughed for the first time in the two and one-half years I had known him.

During the initial phase of the family's therapy, the fathers' interpersonal work with the boy—employing him and supervising him—was the focus of attention. The mother was a guilt-ridden, depressed woman, whose conflicts were worked on during her year of therapy. The father's sensitivity and persistence, coupled with the feedback and encouragement from his group, allowed him to struggle successfully through his son's dilatory tactics and silences. His reward was the slowly decreasing withdrawal and increasing participation of this most difficult patient.

After six months, as the father prepared to leave therapy, he said, "I am in tall cotton. My son is advancing by leaps and bounds—getting new friends, really trying to help himself. He is better today than he was four or five years ago. I am beat. Been with him, thought of him, every minute —day and night." At this time, the mother said in her group, "I feel I am two different people—one at home—maternal, warm, loving; the other —sexy, wild, at the zenith of my sexual powers. I fear you will commit me." At the father's last session in the group, he said, "I learned a lot. I am a happy man. I have not done a lick of work for two weeks—first time in 25 years. I can return to my family."

The mother later reported, "My husband and son now mesh and tangle remarkably. My husband had always let him alone before." She reported that her relationship with her husband had deepened. A frustrated professional woman, gradually unburdened of her heavy load of guilt, she began some refresher courses in her own field. She discontinued therapy eight months later, reporting that the boy was devouring books and happy with the family, though not relating with his peers. He was given permission to audit courses at a top university and later allowed to enroll, leapfrogging over the last year and a half of high school he had missed in his period of decompensation. A few days later, the husband wrote, "Don wishes to see you. The past year has been most rewarding for our family. We seem to have found each other."

Possibly one of those rare and gifted therapists like Frieda Fromm-Reichman or Sechehaye could have achieved some success working with the boy alone. Individual therapy would not, however, have provided the boy with the relationship with his father he so sorely needed.

The family system is the primary focus of attention and effort in this mode of therapy. One therapist alone attempting to influence this complex, built-in arrangement may achieve little success in cases of moderate or great difficulty. The supplemental function of outside groups in defining and strengthening the individual within the family is particularly evident in adolescence, when the peer group adds a necessary element of growth and integration for the individual beyond that which the family can provide. Moreover, therapy groups for each of the parents provide peers who can help them find themselves, accept their shortcomings, and offer means of correcting deficiencies in the family. Acceptance and support of the group, supplementing that from the therapist in the initial stages, ease the need for defensive overreaction in the family.

The therapist, in assigning the participants to therapy groups, is a participant as well as a communications channel joining the individual, his group, and his family. With this approach, each of these factors reinforces the other, since they are interconnected by the supplementary and corrective mechanism which the therapist provides through his personal and technical skills. This arrangement constitutes a synergistic system—that is, the combination is more than the sum of its constituent parts, due to the transactive process and feedback. Since each of these systems converges concurrently, reinforcing the other, the total effect is greater than any individual or system could mobilize alone.

In the middle-class families that I see in my practice, the problem may revolve around an alliance between one parent and the teenager against the other parent, which operates to the detriment of the teenager as well as the parents. It is important to work out the conflicts which prevent one parent from putting the other parent first, so that the individual and relational models the child needs can emerge. This may not be possible in a more serious type of family problem, such as I observed some years ago, where the husband, because of psychosis, alcoholism, and related factors, was unable to fill his role. He was usually unemployed, unwilling to take therapy, and dependent financially on his wife. He procreated children, but did not support them. He was jealous of the children, demanded his wife's complete attention, and was a greater drain on her than any of the children. She could not sustain both, and had to let go of either the children or the husband. It appeared that the wife would do better to divorce her husband.

In an extreme case, the mother, refusing to face the problem with an alcoholic husband who had been repeatedly hospitalized, gave up her adolescent son, who became symptomatic, to foster care and kept a younger, well-behaved child with her. Two years later, when the younger child became an adolescent, the same problem arose again, and the mother again faced the same decision. She let this son go also, rather than commit the husband, who was wearing her down and disturbing the boy.

Another situation was resolved in a more satisfactory way. The 12-year-old daughter of a Mexican migrant farm worker was brought in because of failure at school and behavioral disorders. The family story was as follows. The husband came home once a year in November, got drunk, impregnated his wife, beat her up, took the money she had, and then left. At the time she was seen, she had 10 children. She worked all year to support the children and received nothing from her husband. Her therapy consisted of weekly sessions in a mothers' therapy group. As winter approached, the husband came and went, then the daughter improved. The wife had successfully withstood her husband's demands for the first time and was not pregnant. When the group asked, "Did he not threaten to beat you up?" she replied, "I told him, 'You cannot. I am not alone.' "

Her increased self-esteem and the feeling of support from her group of peers helped her emerge from the bind in which women of her class and culture are often trapped.

SEQUENCE AND DURATION OF THERAPY

Families often ask, "How long does therapy last?" I point out that the initial phase is the evaluation and that the second phase is the achievement of responsibility for self—the understanding and control of one's self and one's functioning in the family and in the group. Some families discontinue therapy with the evaluation or soon after. Others find that after several months the presenting problem is more or less alleviated. At this point some parents may consider that the crisis for which they came no longer exists. They have generally found that it is their repressed conflicts which have prevented the development and growth of their children, but more important, that there has been a non-living area in their own lives—that the energies needed for full growth and enjoyment of life were tied down fruitlessly in unconscious conflict.

A father discontinued therapy connected with an older son, but returned a few years later, when similar problems appeared in the younger son. After a few sessions, he admitted, "Suddenly the problem is not my son anymore. The fight is now between my wife and me." Now, having learned to use the tool of family and group therapy, they faced a decision: did they want to continue to work out the family problems together, or not? The decision was theirs. They knew what the therapy was like, and they knew what they wanted to achieve. In some ways this resembles academic education. One decides how far he wants to go in any area and how much time he wishes to devote to such study.

In the case of one adolescent, Larry, the father found that he had unwittingly adopted the brusque, authoritarian attitude of his own father, against which his son rebelled. He overcame this attitude somewhat as therapy progressed. His wife, at this time, had begun to discover a new freedom for herself, not only in speaking with her husband, but in their sexual relationship, which she was enjoying more. Socially, she found that she had always felt compelled to be the life of the party. She anxiously pressed everyone as she did her son at home. She began to work on this problem. When she felt she had achieved satisfaction in her own relationships, she announced that she, her husband and son were ready to leave therapy. At the next family session, the teenager indicated he did not think the parents were ready to quit. They responded favorably to his suggestion.

Soon thereafter the father discovered that what had caused a low-keyed discordance with his immediate superior—his superior's compulsion to details, faultfinding, and looking over his shoulder—now became an active, painful issue between them. Previously annoyed by this behavior, he now began to find it intolerable. Whereas before he had accumulated such resentment against this man that he feared opening up at all, lest he burst loose completely and lose his job, he now began to talk with his superior in a more rational and effective way, expressing his annoyance. Realizing he unconsciously reacted to his superior as he had to his own father, he gradually achieved a better working relationship. At the subsequent family session, the boy confirmed that his relationship with his father had also improved, and made no objection to his father's discontinuing therapy.

After some months, the mother came in again. A nephew of her husband's, whom she had taken in as a child when his parents died, was very dependent and demanding. She previously tended to disregard him, while compulsively attending to all the amenities of child care. Now she realized her annoyance with him, and faced more openly her feeling of being exploited. She returned to group therapy for a few months, during which time her own dependency needs emerged: reflecting back to her from the child, these caused her annoyance with him. At the same time, she realized more fully how her dependence upon her mother had made her accept many of her mother's manipulative and demanding tactics. She confronted her mother openly, and ultimately the mother came around to accepting her as she was. She now recognized that the symptoms in her adolescent son precipitated a whole chain of action which exposed the conflicting and non-living areas which this family had learned to endure from the past, and incidentally, was passing on to the next generation.

DEVELOPMENT OF FAMILY LEADERSHIP FOR THE ADOLESCENT IN GROUP THERAPY

The therapy group for the adolescent, though not of primary importance, is often an important part of the whole therapy, especially for the older adolescent. At first, the scapegoated "patient's" maladjustment appeared to me to be so overshadowed by the parents' problems that I would not even put the child or the young adolescent into therapy at all. For example, Tom, age 17, had had individual therapy with a child psychiatrist for two and one-half years, but had not improved. The father had been seeing an analyst independently. The returns from these atomistic unrelated efforts were not adequate for this difficult family. Supplementing Tom's and his father's therapy with a therapy group for each and combining this with the therapy of the family as a whole proved more successful in spite of the mother's continued reluctance to become more involved.

I have found that groupings including ages from about 16 years of age to the early 20's are useful, as well as groupings in the narrower age range from 15 to 18. It was gratifying, for example, to see a boy like

Tom, alternately depressed and bored, self-absorbed, anti-everything, interested only in the release he could get from various drugs, gradually open up to the group and show a truly discerning sympathy for a pregnant teenaged girl and an intense commitment to his own family. Parading around in an outlandish getup and in a top hat worn by his grandfather, he was attacked by two teenagers who battered the hat. The deep sadness and grief which he felt revealed his previously concealed feeling for his heritage.

I held a six-hour extended session with his group, to which the adolescents were free to invite their parents. Both Tom and his parents were present at this session. Tom's parents had expressed their anger and anxiety about his coming home late. Choking back his tears, he stated that he himself had been anxious when his parents, who drank heavily, had come home much later than he had expected, for he had feared that they had had an accident. This shaking experience for the parents increased their respect and consideration for him greatly.

It was interesting to watch the adolescents take a turn at leadership in their group. Each exhibited some unusual talent or personality trait. Tom, for example, could draw very well, and brought in some of his surrealistic and symbolic drawings, which provided material for discussion in delving into the unconscious. This stimulated others to bring in their own drawings. Tom's sensitivity and empathy were focused upon as elements with which he could take the leadership in his own family and help his parents in their relationship with him. Thus leadership becomes the inverse of pathology. Tom, for example, could achieve the model for his family, and could convert passivity into activity, frustration and hostility into satisfaction and accomplishment. His growing edge was supported and rewarded in the group. As in football, the group provided the opportunities for scrimmage, practice, and workouts on his problems.

Tom's father in his own group was encouraged to become more assertive with his wife and son, thereby increasing his feeling of self-esteem. This, and increased understanding of his son, also did away with the outbursts of pent-up rage which had alienated and put the son down. This could not very well be accomplished by talking to one person alone.

Group therapy helped prepare Tom for the greater activity and leadership which growth demands, as well as the needs of his problem family. He was able to help motivate his father to accept a more forceful role in the family. The mother, however, came along more slowly. She refused to join a group and attended only occasional family sessions at critical times, "only to help the son."

Parents who cannot relate to a well-functioning therapy group reveal a basic family incapacity. I designate this the "group screen." Like a fluoroscope screen it brings to light otherwise invisible rays. It illuminates and brings into focus elements difficult to discern otherwise. Similarly the group brings to the light of day phenomena that exist unnoticed in the routines of the family. Individual sessions may be required to work through this problem. In this instance a female co-therapist could have helped.

Not only does the leader provide a channel of communication, which he is able to keep open and functioning, but he also has the responsibility of offering a model of acceptance, tolerance, sharing, and communication for the family and its members. When the significant family members have individually accepted responsibility for themselves in the family and their groups, further goals can be clarified with each participant. The function of the group is to support, facilitate, and elicit the unique individuality of each of its members. Conversely, the most significant function of the individual is to be a good group member, to share and make fruitful his uniqueness.

SUMMARY

The principle of synergy is demonstrated by combining family and group therapy modes as a base for adolescent problems the family cannot handle. Individual, family and group sessions are utilized flexibly to this end. Psychological studies reinforce the family evaluation, enabling the significant family members to understand the part each plays in the symptomatic presentation. Each can then actively share in the effort at resolution of the common family problems for himself as well as for the family. Resistances as they occur in any family member need not stop the flow of therapy, since the other members continue with their groups. This prevents escalation of the problem within the family and eases the resolution as information and energy are fed in from other family members and the therapy groups available to them. Examples of vicissitudes and management are given. The interlocking, potentiating combination of group and family therapy is offered as a way of dealing more adequately with more difficult situations.

Especially today, when change and the movement of young people are so prevalent and when change in general is universal, peer group support for the parents, as well as for the adolescents, is essential. The realization of commonality of problems, as well as the development of mutual interests between parents and adolescents, helps bridge the gap which exists in many families.

REFERENCES

BERGER, M., and MENDELL, D. (1967). A preliminary report on participation of patients in more than one psychotherapy group concurrently. *The International Journal of Social Psychiatry,* 13:192-198.

BRUCH, H. (1973). *Eating Disorders: Obesity, Anorexia Nervosa and the Person Within.* New York: Basic Books.

FISHER, S., and MENDELL, D. (1956). Communication of neurotic patterns over two and three generations. *Psychiatry,* 19:41-46.

FISHER, S., and MENDELL, D. (1958). The spread of psychotherapeutic effects from the patient to his family group. *Psychiatry,* 21:133-140.

MENDELL, D., and FISHER, S. (1956). An approach to neurotic behavior in terms of a three generation family model. *The Journal of Nervous and Mental Disease,* 123: 171-180.

MENDELL, D. (1973). Family therapy: A synergistic systems approach. In *Group Therapy 1973,* L. Wolberg and M. Schwartz, eds. New York: Intercontinental Medical Book Corp.

16

Co-Therapists as Advocates in Family Therapy with Crisis-Provoking Adolescents

ROBERT A. SOLOW, M.D. *and*

BEATRICE M. COOPER, M.S.

An old Chinese proverb has it that, "The longer the war continues, the more the enemies look alike." We have found this to be the case in our quest for a peaceful resolution to the warlike crisis which exists in the families of disturbed, provocative adolescents. As co-therapists—a male-female, psychiatrist-social worker team—we have found that the longer the combined psychotherapy continues and the more involved the family members become, the more the former enemies look like friends—familiar aspects of their former selves. This discovery has led us to choose the position, not of peace emissaries, but of advocates.

We have regarded advocacy not as an attempt to fight for the over-powering of one side by the other, nor even as defense, but rather as a way of facilitating better understanding between family members. The co-therapists become the advocates of the whole family, parents and child or children. We are, thus, the defenders of the family and the supporters of all.

The use of co-therapists in family therapy, although relatively new, has already become a useful tool in the armamentarium of those working with families and has been felt by many to be the preferred technique in family therapy (Boszormenyi-Nagy, 1965; Framo, 1962, 1965). Its use as a means of bringing about change in some families with an adolescent member and in catalyzing a developmental trend of those adolescents and parents has been described (Shapiro, 1967). Using this method, some

248

co-therapists have been impressed by the need of the child and of each parent for separation, individualization, and family reintegration experiences (Belmont and Jasnow, 1961).

In our joint work, we treat the adolescent who has threatened his or her family's structure by involving all the family members in a crisis situation. We have found it useful to involve the adolescent patient in individual psychotherapeutic treatment with the psychiatrist who, concurrently and in conjunction with the social worker, is a co-therapist and advocate for the family and the teenager in conjoint family therapy. Our patients have been adolescents whose precipitating incident has come to a point of crisis, often with the overdosage of drugs. These adolescents have been involved in the past in other methods of treatment which have failed, as have their attempts at some separation from their family. The parents have responded to the sudden confrontation with their child's—heretofore hidden—acting-out behavior with desperation, confusion, and shock. Although presented with subtle or overt evidence of this behavior before the crisis, these parents were unable to cope with the symptomatic evidence and needed to disbelieve it and to feel that nothing was amiss.

As professional colleagues in private practice, we have pooled our individual resources, discipline, and training. By so doing, we have found our efforts more effectively successful even in cases where past individual therapy alone had failed. In arriving at the formulation of this technique we were aware that we already knew how to mobilize ourselves to deal with an entry at a point of crisis. We could recognize that the crisis was usually a critical time in a young person's life in that he had finally succeeded in calling his parents' attention to his festering and cumulative need for help.

Working with these parents stimulated insights into our own past, made us question our own value system, the relationship of generations, and the meaning of maturation. We began to feel that the old ways were not always effective. Although we were not seeking a new way of working, we modified and adapted our known ways to get immediately into the critical situation so that a family could reflect and enter into a genuine therapeutic alliance. We recognized that if we did not have the opportunity to work on the acting out of such a life-and-death drama, we would never be able to understand better how this desperate situation came about. Actually, we were pragmatists because, while we wanted an opportunity to do the work we had confidence in doing, we were not sure we could do it unless we first did something about the immediate crisis.

We began, as so many have done, by listening to parents pressuring us for an immediate appointment. Often referred by the internist who had saved the life of the child from an overdose of drugs, the parent, usually the mother, either at the doctor's office or in the emergency room, pleaded with the psychiatrist to be seen immediately. Even while doing so, she was simultaneously reassuring him that this child had never presented problems before and had never given any evidence of being troubled or unhappy. It would appear that the parents could cope with the extent of the problem only by deceiving themselves, by denying that anything had troubled their child previously. Thus, we began with the urgent telephone call from the parents who, while vigorously denying any previous history of difficulties, aggressively demanded not only an *immediate appointment,* but also an *immediate solution.* It was an extension of what we had been experiencing in this particular generation—instant remedies for all society's ills.

Later in the process, the social worker was introduced to the family to obtain a more comprehensive picture of its members and history. The parents continued to maintain massive denial even as they began to reveal the underlying terror they had been experiencing during the long germination of the present episode. We began our advocatory function by appealing to the parents to allow the child to be in treatment.

We found our method suitable for adolescents in individual treatment who were not able to function in the family without creating severe crisis. We did not delineate the roles for the co-therapists, nor plan any long-range strategy in advance, except as it evolved out of the transference in the family therapy sessions with the parents. We recognized the danger of overidentification and countertransference feelings towards a particular family member (Belmont and Jasnow, 1961; Arlen, 1966; Rubinstein and Weiner, 1967), but discussed this before and after the sessions in order to be cognizant of our individual response to the therapy process. As did Johnson and Szurek (1952), we recognized that collaborative therapists must be uncompetitive, unambivalent, and cooperative with each other.

As co-therapists who had worked together on many cases over a long period of time, we found that we frequently arrived at certain insights simultaneously. We had to be aware of meaningful ways we could reinforce each other without overwhelming the family members or creating a dichotomy between those who got help and those who gave help. We needed to guard against revealing our mutual independent insight so that the patients themselves could arrive at meaningful insights.

In another communication (Solow and Cooper, 1974) we described how, with this approach, we could rapidly form a therapeutic alliance. Instead of a shortcut, in many ways this approach was more intensive than the individual approach. We described, in that article, how each member of the family became involved, focusing immediately on the implication of the use of denial and its meaning by the family, and how the drug-oriented girls evoked specific feelings in their fathers. We observed that, initially, the adolescent patients resisted the tie to the father figure, and that both father and daughter maintained an unconscious denial concerning the extensiveness of the pathology and the use of drugs. With the introduction of the co-therapist technique, the adolescent girls used the psychiatrist as a confidant, pouring out extensive material revealing their pathology. They put the psychiatrist in the somewhat helpless and exceedingly difficult position of knowing all but being powerless to use this material in any kind of protective, direct way. The psychiatrist, understanding the dynamics, could not risk or undermine the basic trust which the patient had bestowed upon him. Yet this trust rendered him as helpless as the father had been at the point of beginning the treatment process.

We understood that this kind of transference condition is one in which the psychiatrist became the all-understanding, but powerless, father figure with whom the girl began to build a close relationship. It takes tremendous skill to maintain this condition and makes the social worker, who is then conjointly working with the parents both individually and in the family therapy sessions, the recipient of the negative transference of the adolescent patient. One adolescent became furious with the social worker for an interpretation and said, "Why don't you shut your mouth? How come all of a sudden my parents are suspicious, questioning, checking?" This teenager had been planning to participate in a peace vigil in one of the local parks, a ruse for getting high on drugs and openly engaging in sexual intercourse. It had been presented differently to the mother, whom the social worker had subtly encouraged to raise some questions, thereby revealing the hidden purpose behind the request to participate.

Frequently, an adolescent would look directly at the social worker while blatantly lying or distorting his requests. Eventually the patient recognized the wish to be found out, the struggle to tell the truth, and the need to gratify the impulse, and thus to lie. When this material was revealed, the psychiatrist would then help the patient to understand his own behavior.

The social worker would attempt to help the parents work through their need to deny, and begin to become more active, strong parents, with the capacity to understand what their child was doing without becoming punitive.

We saw in our families a particular phenomenon which deviates from the usual kind of family structure in which individuals use work as an organizing principle. Ordinarily, when people become parents, work and family life are the organizing principles, so that parents become vulnerable to their children's developmental difficulties. They feel they have failed if their child does not satisfactorily negotiate each successive stage of development. We have examined what causes parents to react to illnesses in the child, their reality and their own personality problems. We have recognized that there is a back-and-forth, and/or combination of the symbiotic and the autistic positions in the adolescent's relation to the parents; as they negotiate to separate, they choose pathological means.

The current understanding suggests that children have existence and identity of their own, apart from, although related to, the parents in the family. Erikson's writings (1968) have carefully demonstrated each of the developmental stages the child goes through in relation to himself, to his parents, and to the family. The children we have seen have chosen to bring difficulties in experiencing themselves as vital, active people into the combination of individual and family therapy. They have helpless egos and are passively overwhelmed by demands from id, superego, or reality pressure. Our work has concerned not just "the cause of illness," but has rather been directed primarily to "the cause of the cure" (Ekstein and Friedman, 1972). While the adolescents we have seen are creating conflicts in their task of finding objects outside the parental figures towards whom to direct their libidinal strivings, they seem to be struggling with conflicts derived from much earlier periods of development.

Following the discovery of the event to which the whole family was reacting, its members frequently said they were unaware that the child was troubled, that they presumed the communication that existed was ideal, and that things were going fairly well. Our format was usually to have the child seen initially by the psychiatrist, while the social worker usually had the initial contact with the parents. Within this structure we found that the adolescent child revealed far more pathology than the parents ever dreamed existed. The parents, striving to maintain an image of themselves as understanding and tolerant, would suddenly panic and become restrictive by denying freedom to the child at a time when the child really needed fewer restrictions. Thus the child frequently got a double message: "We approve, but we don't approve." The explosion came as a complicated outgrowth of a situation in which the parents permitted too much freedom; the parents overreacted to the event with too much control and restriction; the child began treatment with the psychiatrist by bitterly complaining about how strict the parents were now that he had been honest with them about his problems.

The adolescent usually expressed his protest at this point with words such as, "I can control myself now. I have learned my lesson, I want to live my own life. If this is the way it's going to be, I might as well run away." Or, very commonly, "I can't wait until I'm 18 to move out." In most of these situations we found the adolescent girl had a very loyal boy friend who understood her, with whom she maintained a secret alliance, and with whom she wanted to run away to escape a potentially intolerable situation in the parental home. The parents frequently assumed the attiude, "It's a phase—is it really a problem?" In order to maintain a kind of naïveté, they needed to be deceived, because they had idealized their family life and actually believed that they had been communicating by being so permissive and so free. They needed to feel deceived because they were afraid of what might be revealed without the deception. Consequently, they maintained stronger and stronger denials of any "real" difficulty even while behaving very rigidly, sometimes to the point of physically restricting the child to the premises.

To illustrate, for over four months 15-year-old Sally had been taking her parents' car in the middle of the night for a tryst with a boy friend, and then returning the car to the garage and going back to bed. The parents, unusually light sleepers who ordinarily had trouble maintaining their sleep with the ordinary residential neighborhood noises, never heard a sound during their daughter's nocturnal activities. Nor did they make anything of her progressively increasing sleepiness and deterioration in school performance. Even when they were told by a neighbor that she had been seen out at night they chose not to believe it until, indeed, one morning the father had to go to work especially early and discovered she was missing. They responded by restricting her to her room after school and on weekends, nailing the windows shut, and practically standing guard to prevent her departure.

In such a situation, the adolescent protests and presents the constant threat "to split" from the family rather than effect a process of separation.*

In our approach, simultaneous with the diagnostic evaluation the child was given psychological tests. With this we observed another phenomenon which clinicians find puzzling. Some parents do not want to know the results of the psychological tests which point out dynamics and propensities for acting out. Some parents will agree to the child's being in treatment but will resist the inclusion of other family members, insisting that the problem is just a small one that can be dealt with between the child and the psychiatrist. We learned the hard way not to reveal anything about the psychological testing to the parents unless the child was included in the family session, and then, only enough to enable the child to have an honest confrontation with what he inwardly knew to be his problem. The child frequently used the psychological tests in order to convince the parents of the need for ongoing treatment. Sometimes the parents preferred to manipulate a solution to the problem by attempting to legislate procedures for the child's behavior. They demanded a separation from the peer group which was allegedly a bad influence, restricted friends' coming and going, proposed moving away from the community—everything in order to isolate the adolescent from "peer contamination." One mother took her daughter to the beach, managed to get some distance between them, and then used binoculars in order to observe her behavior. Later she asked her daughter what she had been doing in the time they were separated.

In this phase of the treatment program, parents usually devised artificial superego strength as if to fill in the superego lacunae (Johnson and Szurek, 1952) with putty and seal them off. They could thus pretend that if they were firm and overly controlling, they could prevent anything from happening, though they ignored the developmental processes that go on within each individual. At this point, in their work with the social worker, the parents began to find that external solutions were their des-

---

* In the studies conducted by McGregor and associates (1964), they presented a method of helping a family grow as it confronted the crisis of its adolescent members, using the team therapy approach in which therapists of various disciplines worked together. Although they worked within a very short and extremely limited time structure, they soon recognized that patterns of parental interaction were apt to produce and maintain in dynamic equilibrium specific forms of developmental arrest in the offspring. They also recognized that certain types of interaction in the teamwork itself, as well as in the family, could serve as a model of behavior for the family's identifying with problem-solving experts. The team felt that they served as a model for healthy group functioning and made channels of communication easier.

perate attempts to be superb manipulators, but they could not ignore the internal processes, the forces that worked within each of them. In an educational and intellectual way, as the *child's* advocate, we tried then to help the parents separate what was really appropriate from what was inappropriate for this phase of development.

We know that we prepare the latency child for adolescence by trusting, although not blindly trusting. Frequently parents began to observe that what they had seen and accepted as evidence of good behavior and indices of normal development had been bizarre. One mother's so-called proof as to how competently she and her daughter had handled presentation of menstruation was that the child gaily danced around with her sanitary belt and napkin outside her jeans. Another parent tried to explain her child's overdose of drugs with barbiturates as something that every adolescent does at one time or another. Thus, the social worker had to unscramble distortions to help the parents distinguish between and deal with age-appropriate and age-inappropriate behavior. We also observed that parents edited versions of the events so that we were immediately confronted with two sets of facts—revised and actual. Some of the material which emerged within the presence of the family was devastating, as in the situation with the above-mentioned Sally.

She had been belligerent when the parents had finally confronted her with their outrage at her taking out the family car in the middle of the night. She cried as she confessed meeting her boy friend, a convicted felon, for protection from her adopted older brother who had been seducing her for months. These parents responded with shame and guilt when they found themselves angrily behaving exactly like their own parents decades before. The father's expression of his bitter feelings, at present towards the adopted son and in the past towards his own father, enabled him to become generally more fatherly towards his frightened 15-year-old daughter. She began to feel his empathy instead of being frightened off by his protectiveness. Eventually this change in awareness led to the family's ability to recognize that the adopted son had severe problems for which he needed long, intensive, individual therapy.

We thought that the symptomatology of our young patients indicated their means of struggling to effect some kind of individuation which their parents were psychologically unable to accept. In these families, the problem was not one of poor communication, but rather of faulty communication. It had developed because the need to deceive and to be deceived had been chosen as a way of allowing beginning separation. The faultiness of the method, however, perpetuated poor impulse control and over-closeness to parents.

Sue, 15½ years old, was seen in consultation after her emergency hospitalization because of an overdose of tranquilizers and sleeping pills. This girl was devious enough, and the parents' unconscious denial strong enough, that the parents had been unaware of her drug experiences and of any sexual experiences she had had while under the influence of the drugs. The parents, seen together, were furious because they saw their daughter as dishonest, unworthy, and manipulative. Both of them saw their child as the damaged part of themselves and felt that she genetically carried insanity. Although she did not know the details of what had gone on in the individual contact between Sue and the psychiatrist, the social worker's subtle intervention in the family sessions enabled the parents to break through their need to believe that things had been stabilized. The revelation of game playing and breaking through the denial in the family session permitted the adolescent to experience her parents as protective, concerned, and non-intrusive. In turn, the parents rather than behaving punitively as had been their accustomed response, tried to make themselves available and constructively helpful. For example, a crisis had developed when Sue loaned her car to a friend who crashed it.

The parents had retaliated by taking away the car and the patient had had temper tantrums. The parents were angry at Sue who, they felt, was not making any progress nor doing the things she should be doing. In the family session they set out to attack her. Both the psychiatrist and the social worker became advocates for the child. While the psychiatrist supported the child's positive qualities, the social worker attempted to hold the parents to the goals of separation and responsibility that had been previously set for the child. The girl had telephoned her mother to advise her in advance that she wished to loan her car to this unnamed friend. In the mother's desire to help, she had not directly discussed the whole question with her daughter, who was hinting at the nature of the relationship with her friend. In retrospect, the mother recognized she had evaded her own responsibilities and had encouraged her daughter's "motherliness" with peers. She appreciated her daughter's sensitivity and her willingness to help them in times of trouble, such as substituting for them in their jobs, baby-sitting for their siblings, and cooking and cleaning for their working, single-parent mothers. She accepted Sue as an adequate, whole person outside of the home, but within the home situation, the mother felt threatened. There, she saw Sue as a competitor for her husband as well as a more competent, more affectionate, younger mother with the baby brother. Whenever Sue's activities outside the home led to difficulties with the father, the mother kept her distance in order to permit the father to attack Sue physically through beatings.

In the family sessions we observed how Sue invited the social worker both to protect her and to discover her outside involvements, while at the same time wanting the psychiatrist "to rip into her." When this was painfully repeated, the parents wept because they had created such a masochistic pattern within their family. They were able to see that Sue wanted not a sexual involvement with the father, but a protective, tender, parental relationship. She knew no way to get it other than to invite suspicion. This understanding led to her insight into her lack of trust in anyone and her feeling that anyone permitted to know her really well would not be able to tolerate her. As she revealed her deep sense of unworthiness and despair at being unable to have a close relationship with anyone, the mother began to notice a change in their relationship. She and Sue became more spontaneous with each other and more sharing. The father recognized his contribution to the family dilemma: he had behaved in an overcontrolling, overdirective manner and had not permitted Sue to have a close relationship with her mother whom he judged as weak and ineffectual; he had regarded his wife as a cold, superficial, uninvolved individual like his mother and thus had felt it was mandatory for him to assume both parental roles.

On occasions, the psychiatrist, in his role as advocate, interceded for the parents and the social worker could switch her role to plead for increased responsibility for the teenager. Thus the co-therapist-advocate roles were not rigid or restricted but could vary for the benefit of any family members involved in the treatment. In Martha's situation, when the father was away on business (a frequent occurrence), the mother would abdicate her role as parent and join the children in defying the family structure. While the father was away, Martha felt helpless and abandoned, and provoked increased crisis with drugs and sexual acting out. When the mother telephoned the father for support, he would react to her with helplessness and rage for making things more difficult while he was preoccupied with business. Once when the father was away, Martha, her sister, and mother were seen together in the family session. They all then revealed that they were afraid of the father's rage and/or silence.

The three women of the family hoped that when the father returned to the family sessions after his trip, the co-therapists would plead their case for them. They asked us to be their advocates in helping the father accept them the way they really were, not the way he thought they were. They wanted him to see them as friends, not enemies—to end the war. At the same time, the therapist tried to help the mother recognize the predicament in which she was placing the helpers. In the past when father returned home, he reprimanded his wife for her irresponsibility and inadequate care for the children and made Martha "daddy's pet." Instead of being confronted with the crisis caused by her behavior, she saw it projected on to her mother who consequently suffered her husband's fury. He became distant, uncommunicative, and unloving. The parents, who anticipated reunions as occasions to enjoy sexual gratification, would generally find that the consequence of Martha's actions was the creation of an obstacle to such behavior.

Following the father's return home, there were frequent sessions in which Martha pointed out how her mother's neglect had made her vulnerable to being tempted to take drugs. The mother then wondered why Martha was trying to sabotage the relationship between the parents. The psychiatrist helped the family recognize the connection between the father's absence and its effect on everyone in the family.

Martha, in an unconscious bid for attention, would invariably become involved in an accident and so evoke only sympathy and kindness from her father. As a result, his reunion with his wife became a stormy battle. The father, anxious over each separation from his family, frequently became depressed as he was about to leave and terminated each departure with explosive, silent withdrawal. The mother, resentful because of his leaving her, of the responsibility for sole care of the family, and of the necessity to carry out the orders he left behind, was unable to express her longing for her husband and sadness at being separated from him. Instead, she fantasied the good times he was having and became increasingly tearful and unassured. Meanwhile, when not engaged in his business activities, the father actually sat alone in his hotel room, fantasying his "ideal" family and how to make contact with them. However, as the time for reunion approached, he would think about the responsibilities he had placed upon the mother, would be anxious about the bad news she might have phoned him or which might be awaiting him, and would arrive home worried and questioning.

Gradually this family developed the capacity to deal with their feelings about abandonment and separation from each other. In one session, mother commented that there were only two people in the world she could depend on—a neighbor who cared for her, and herself. As she succinctly put it, "When all the chips are down, who do I have? Nobody." The father's response was one of overwhelming sadness to what was a terrible accusation. Yet, he had never told his wife he loved her, nor had the children ever felt that he cared for their mother. The children were deeply affected by this spontaneous revelation. They felt that their mother should know they loved her, that they would care if something happened to her. This led to their admission that, like their father, they believed that the open expression of tender feelings could lead to loss and damage. The father saw the expression of tenderness and of needing another person as tremendously damaging. He used his family in a very punitive way. He called his wife dreadful names and repeatedly threatened her. But he never saw this kind of behavior as damaging or harmful to his family. In this situation, the co-therapists were advocates for the whole family.

As the individual members of the family developed a transference towards the psychiatrist, they began to accept their positive feelings toward the father figure. This was countered for a time by their attitude towards the social worker. In the waiting room the mother and daughters would ridicule the social worker; they were frequently sarcastic and denigrating about her. Yet in the actual therapy session, they would look directly to her for approval. On the other hand, the father developed a positive transference to the social worker. When he felt he was ready to withdraw from the family sessions, he responded positively in a meeting with the social worker, showing trust and respect. Soon afterwards, the mother began overtly to identify with the social worker. She showed care in her grooming and appearance and confessed her earlier feelings of competitiveness and resentment towards "the other woman."

The psychiatrist went on vacation to the Middle East at a time when many planes were being hijacked. When the family sessions resumed, the father confessed his concern about the psychiatrist's safe return. By then, the entire family was better able to deal directly with their longing for tenderness and more affectionate relationships with one another. Significantly, these parents became more sensitive to their aging parents' problems, which in the past had caused considerable turmoil in the home. The children, who had been competitive when the grandparents became ill, were appalled at their own unexpressed death wishes towards the grandparents. As their relationship with their parents improved, however, they could allow their parents to become parental figures towards the dying grandparents without feeling threatened. We felt this was an index of progressive development of a greater ego integration, which enabled the children to function more independently and more competently on their own.

We were able to work with this family until Martha was 18 and moved out of the home. Previously she had threatened to do this in a way that created tremendous anxiety for herself and her parents. When the actual time came, she and a girl friend moved into an apartment on the property of a faculty member from a nearby university. Her dream of dropping out, becoming a hippie, and living out of a Volkswagen bus was appropriately converted into something more conducive to further ego development.

SUMMARY

In order to paraphrase the Chinese proverb which suggests that a prolonged war makes enemies look more and more alike, we need to stress a process of helping which is based on having each therapist who works with one member of the family become also the advocate of the other. In such a situation the process will produce a solution in which the differences between the generations will be synthesized more and more by a common denominator, family unity and shared family interests. The adolescent struggle towards separation, instead of turning toward pathological rebellion, will turn into an individuation process supported by the parents who cease to be threatened by it. Perhaps the function of family advocacy can lead, in many cases, to the realization of the *bon mot* by Mark Twain: "When I was 14 I thought my father was stupid. When I became 20 I was surprised by how much he had learned in so very few years."

REFERENCES

ARLEN, M. S. (1966). Conjoint therapy and the corrective emotional experience. *Family Process*, 5:91-104.

BELMONT, L. P., and JASNOW, A. (1961). The utilization of co-therapists and of group therapy techniques in a family-oriented approach to a disturbed child. *International Journal of Group Psychotherapy*, 11:319-328.

BOSZORMENYI-NAGY, I. (1965). Intensive family therapy as process. In *Intensive Family Therapy: Theoretical and Practical Aspects*. I. Boszormenyi-Nagy and J. L. Framo, eds., pp. 87-142. New York: Harper & Row.

EKSTEIN, R., and FRIEDMAN, S. (1972). *The Challenge: Despair and Hope in the Conquest of Inner Space*. New York: Brunner/Mazel.

ERIKSON, E. H. (1968). *Identity, Youth and Crisis*. New York: Norton.

FRAMO, J. L. (1962). The theory of the technique of family treatment of schizophrenia. *Family Process*, 11:119-131.

FRAMO, J. L. (1965). Rationale and technique of intensive family therapy. In *Intensive Family Therapy: Theoretical and Practical Aspects*, I. Boszormenyi-Nagy and J. L. Framo, eds., pp. 143-212. New York: Harper & Row.

JOHNSON, A. M., and SZUREK, S. A. (1952). The genesis of antisocial acting out in children and adults. *Psychoanalytic Quarterly*, 21:323-343.

McGREGOR, R., RITCHIE, A. M., SERRANO, A. C., SCHUSTER, F. P., MacDONALD, E. C., and GOLISHIAN, H. A. (1964). *Multiple Impact Therapy with Families*. New York: McGraw-Hill.

RUBINSTEIN, D., and WEINER, O. R. (1967). Co-therapy teamwork relations in family psychotherapy. In *Family Therapy and Disturbed Families*, G. H. Zuk and I. Boszormenyi-Nagy, eds., pp. 206-219. Palo Alto: Science and Behavior Books.

SHAPIRO, R. G. (1967). The origin of adolescent disturbances in the family. In *Family Therapy and Disturbed Families*. G. H. Zuk and I. Boszormenyi-Nagy, eds. Palo Alto: Science and Behavior Books.

SOLOW, R. A., and COOPER, B. M. (1974). Therapeutic mobilization of families around drug-induced adolescent crises. *Adolescent Psychiatry*. Vol. III, Sherman C. Feinstein and Peter L. Giovacchini, eds. New York: Basic Books.

17

The Use of Multiple Family Therapy
Groups with Adolescent Drug Addicts

DORIS BARTLETT, M.A.

The primary purpose of this chapter is to report on the use of multiple family therapy with addicted adolescents from an urban ghetto.

A brief sketch is necessary to provide a framework for understanding some of the shaping forces in the lives of these young people and their families. The parents in the families we worked with were, for the most part, Spanish-speaking immigrants, and poor black and white "hard-core" ghetto-dwellers; many of them had been trapped in the slums for the past 15 or 20 years. Very few families were intact. They had at least twice as many people as the living space was meant to accomodate. Often the shabby, ancient, fragile tenement apartments would have a costly barricade erected for protection of the one possession of value—the TV.

The street life is dangerous and surfeited with mean sights and smells. The school life, determined by worn-out, often frightened teachers and by an arid curriculum, remote from the life being lived, contains little joy or learning. First and second graders are already being shifted or even "expelled" as incorrigible. The difficulties of teaching and learning to read in these schools are notorious. Their atmosphere vibrates with mutual suspicion, fear and hostility. Failure in school is more common than success for these adolescents and children.

The art of survival must be exquisitely fashioned by the young, poor minority member and his family in an urban ghetto existence. Skill and know-how are required to understand, negotiate and circumvent the entangling systems of housing, education, welfare, as well as the subsystems of street gangs, drug pushers, organized and disorganized crime. The deprivations, economic and personal, do not allow for a solid sense of worth and self-esteem, but can make for an *overwhelming sense of insignificance*. Those who do not master the necessary skills seek other means of coping with these tasks of survival. Eventually, for some, the "drug-scene" may appear to offer a solution whereby the world seems enlarged, failures and conflicts minimized. "Spacing-out" can provide a *sense* of mastery and relieve an overloaded family life and individual psychic apparatus.

Turmoil in the lives of these children does not start at adolescence; it is integral to the chaotic family and neighborhood life that forms the chrysalis from which these adolescents emerge. Of necessity a ghetto family requires of the children early quasi-independence and self-reliance, plus language skills to help the family through the confusing networks of local institutions. Adult-like responsibilities and responses to crises are thrust upon the youngsters, and yet there is an overt expectation of unquestioning obedience to parental authority. The rules are vague, often inappropriate to the immediate milieu and impossible to enforce, at times capricious and arbitrary, derived from some momentary necessity or harassment felt by the parent. Modes of communication frequently create confusion rather than clarification for the children. Shifts in the power structure occur early in the life cycle of the families. In the frustration growing out of their own unmet external and internal needs, the parents feel helpless and affectionally needy, and often abdicate. The pain in their lives is expressed through unalleviated depressions, or vague, but incapacitating, physical ailments and hopelessness. When, in viewing this group, we consider the adolescent's need for self-differentiation and autonomy, the questions arise: autonomy from whom? and when? As Minuchin et al. (1967) state, "the siblings become the socializers, interpreters, the moralistic pack and the rescue squad." They also suggest that in such families the development of differentiation and autonomy may have to be evaluated on the basis of "response-appraisal" from siblings and peers rather than from parents.

Turmoil is also reflected in the lack of "orderly" development in these children. Auerswald (1964) in his discussion of the cognitive development of children attending a health clinic in a ghetto points out that "they demonstrate a lack of differentiating capacities for time, space or role change in response to different people; they lack a sense of mastery or the ability to plan and anticipate events . . . and find meaning in life only within the immediate family. . . . The emotions they experience are related to individual survival—fear, rage and sexual sensation."

Though many of the adolescents with whom we worked demonstrated in their earlier years both the precocity and deficiencies described by Auerswald (1964) (substantiated by the author's experience with psychological evaluations of the same population), somehow the cognitive skills related to survival techniques and coping with life are not measured. Nor are the addict's skills for buying, selling, traveling, or the overall ability to "hustle" tapped as potentials in schools or guidance centers in preadolescence.

The familiar concepts of superego lacunae, suffusion of id impulses or oral fixations do not adequately explain either the precocities or the deficiencies in these children, *and may obscure the realities of the familial and social contexts of their development*. They suffer all kinds of lacunae. The more middle-class youngster who starts to deal in drugs and is addicted frequently claims he is simply imitating "business." Even with these young people to talk of super-ego lacunae begs the question when we have only to read of Watergate. At such times it is no longer a matter of lacunae, but of a "norm." The point here is that an unacknowledged norm does exist for ghetto-raised people; it is used by professionals frequently and mechanically, the base standard being adaptations to middle-class ideals in education and intellectual matters, ethics and psycho-social development. However, the content of more or less healthy adaptations can be interpreted differently, based on class background. The phenomena of boredom, for instance, and the search for a "high" are different when they are a means of coping with an overabundance of food, commodities and parental indulgences and the role of being an object of display for parental success, than when they are a means of coping with deprivations, the inundations of erratic, disparate, confusing stimuli in street and home, and the role of being a burden.

Consequently, for the adolescent addict in the ghetto, societal and familial dysfunctions emerge as dominant influences in fostering addiction, even in altering the "normal" intrapsychic development. If the adolescent remains within the family the addiction will be found to be syntonic with some aspect of the family functioning. (It is, obviously, syntonic with certain practices and values within the larger social milieu.) With these young people it is of particular importance to draw other members of the family into the therapy on the assumption that drug addiction in family members could be understood as a symptom of family interactional and transactional difficulties (Framo, 1970).

Drug addiction does appear to be a versatile symptom since it has the qualities of an epidemiological, yet mystifying, disease. It can be a prominent topic of concern and of warnings within the family while it remains shrouded in its own cult, jargon and rituals. It can have the convenience of a foregone conclusion ("we knew this would happen") or be maintained as a "family secret" that aids in obscuring other disturbances.

The decision to use multiple family therapy (MFT) as a primary mode of treatment was based on the reports of Laqueur (1964, 1972; Laqueur et al., 1969). Although MFT began as an expedient measure to deal with large numbers of schizophrenic patients in a state hospital, it was soon found to shorten the time of therapy. Conflictual family situations were reproduced with less anxiety in the presence of other families and therapists than in individual or single family sessions. Laqueur (1964) believes that this occurs because MFT provides a setting for learning by analogy, identification with, and imitation of other families' healthier modes and styles, and through the therapists' adroit use of various participants in specific co-therapy roles and the skillful manipulation of competition.

Clearly the life-style of the family contributes to the emergence of the addicted adolescent. Therefore we considered change in the family mode essential to planning for rehabilitation. We were also faced with the problem of large numbers, a meager staff and too little time.

The following describes family treatment in two discrete settings which are contiguous and deal with the same population at different points in time—a detoxification program and a residential treatment program. Patients from the former frequently elected the latter after detoxification. The groups described are addicted adolescents and their families, addicted adolescent couples, and a group of parents of adolescent addicts in residential treatment.

MULTIPLE FAMILY THERAPY IN A SHORT-TERM HOSPITAL DETOXIFICATION PROGRAM

In this group our aim was to intervene at a *point of possible change,* induced by the crisis that precipitated the decision for detoxification, the detoxification process itself and the institutional pressures for relinquishing drugs.

The patients were primarily heroin addicts, although the number of multidrug abuses and lethal combinations of methadone and alcohol was increasing. The age range reported here is from 15 to 21. The drug abuse or addiction dated from one to eight years. Two-thirds were from the lowest economic level and the rest from the blue-collar level and lower middle class. These patients came from local and suburban ghetto areas around the city (though an increasing number were from wealthier suburbs).

Admission to the hospital is voluntary: thus any patient in the "detox" program could leave before the end of the three-weeks' stay provided. The expectation (hope) of the staff was that the patients would remain at least until they were medically "clean." The overall program included helping the patients with welfare, court and probation systems, arranging for and escorting patients to special clinics when necessary, and maintaining a flow of activity on the wards. The thrust of the ward counseling was directed toward the future, toward helping the patient come to a decision to relinquish or control the addiction by accepting a drug-free or methadone program.

Our goals for the family therapies were:

(a) educating the family to the role of the detoxification program and the need to plan for rehabilitation;
(b) examining the family relationships to determine what deterrents and attributes existed that could affect planning;
(c) helping families help one another to cope with the shame and helplessness often related to having a young addict in the family;
(d) planning for rehabilitation by enlisting family cooperation;
(e) helping the family find alternative ways to cope with conflicts that obstructed cooperation.

Patients were referred by ward counselors who became increasingly sensitive to troublesome family relationships; much depended on the counselor's ability to discern a "family problem." We stipulated that the patient, not the counselor, was required to contact the family members. We regarded the willingness to do this as a crude measure of motivation to engage in family treatment.

We accepted as "family" people with whom the patient *lived and had emotional ties.* This often resulted in the attendance of a homosexual partner, or a recently acquired common-law spouse, a friend, a neighbor, or a cousin. We tried to exclude those who made it blatantly obvious they were there to visit or were a security threat (i.e. maneuvering to smuggle drugs into the ward).

The emphasis on family interviews as part of treatment created some controversy and doubt among the staff, particularly since there was little published material at the time that was convincing. The effort was considered questionable for detoxification patients, expressed as, "our patients don't want to bother with their families at such a time," or "the families were simply relieved that the patient was out of the way." However, within a four-month period we proliferated from one MFT group to three. The patients were responsive, perhaps in proportion to the enthusiasm of the staff. When it was recognized that this was not a panacea for addiction there was a leveling off of interest. Staff members who could accept the limitations of four to six sessions remained with the effort. The number of sessions was determined by the fact that there were no funds available for an aftercare program; the work had to be done within the hospitalization period.

CHARACTERISTICS OF THE MFT AND COUPLES' GROUPS

Usually the sessions were attended by an average of four families, two therapists and a "participant-observer." The therapists were drawn from the professional and paraprofessional staff who were able to give evening time.

A typical group could consist of three adolescent addicts (15 to 19 years old, male or female), a parent or both parents, usually one or two siblings, an older patient and a marital partner or relative. The patients were brought down from the wards by one therapist while the other brought the family members in from the waiting area. The sessions were held in the evening for an hour and a half, and met once a week, except for an inpatient couples group which met twice a week.

The leaders started by welcoming the family members, explaining their goals to the group and trying to lead into the question of rehabilitation. In this stage the family usually made it clear that "there were no problems before the addiction." "We are a very close family, we love one another, the only trouble is the drugs," etc. An extreme of this stance was evident in one family of four, *all* of whom were in the hospital for detoxification at the same time—Mrs. P., age 38; Raymond, age 19; Grace, age 18; and Marie, a cousin, age 18. The son, as spokesman for the family affirmed: "We *really* love, uh, because we feel for one another. We have know-how to take care . . . when one ODs. We help each other . . . sister puts out, I make the connections . . . and mother prepares the stuff. We're here because the drug [cocaine] is bad . . . for the mind, and for the teeth." (He had lost most of his teeth.)

During the first session certain strategies were common and readily identifiable: complaints about the limited nature of the detoxification program by parents or spouse; patients sending the message, "It's bad here, boring; I'm suffering"; relatives showing concern and directing questions to the therapists about proper medications. Another strategy was the in-group drug talk, eliciting the interest, fascination and *silence* of the family members not involved with drugs. Often this triggered competition among the families to establish a position of superiority either through avowed innocence or great knowledge of the drug scene. The themes related to trust, blame, willpower, and disavowal of knowledge of the addiction.

Excerpt from a First Session

This group was attended by the A.s—Jean the patient, age 19 and her widowed father; the P.s described above; the L.s—Pat, age 18, and her mother, also a widow in her middle years; and the R.s—Vi, age 17, her sister, age 19, and her mother, who was separated from the father. Mrs. R. has two other younger children who did not attend the sessions. Pat has a child who was placed in a foster home by the courts. Before she could have her child back Pat needed to be drug-free on a methadone program for a year! Jean had been "on her own" since her mother died four years previously. She had no siblings or close relations.

The P.s had expressed, through Raymond, some shame that their whole family had become addicted to heroin; they were less so when they learned that one of Pat's brothers had died a year ago of an overdose. Raymond tells his family that he is in the process of deciding to go to Phoenix or Sera (residential treatment programs). Mrs. P. seems vaguely aware of what he has said, but his sister and cousin accept his statements with skeptical, knowing shrugs, implying that they had heard it all before. Raymond says, "I'm the man, the head of the family . . . it's up to me . . . this time I'm gonna do it. . . ."

Suddenly Jean screams at her father in excellent Brooklynese: "You lousy drunk, you were wet for 30 years. It killed my mother, and you lookin' down your nose at *me*! Whadd'ya ever do for me, huh? You gonna come roun' here and tell *me*! . . . the goddam nerve!"

Meanwhile, prim Mrs. L., her eyebrows up and her back very straight, turns to *her* daughter, whose smile and giggle betray appreciation of Jean's tirade, and says: "Well, I mean, Pat, *you* didn't have that kind of trouble . . . you had a good home . . . but nothing ever pleased you. I don't mean to criticize. . . . I mean, dear, I know this time you're going to make it . . . but maybe it was because you lost father and always managed to get your own way . . . that's why you turned to using . . . uh . . . you know."

The two therapists look around this group and hope someone will ask Mrs. L. what she means by "you know," but know that this ignorance or delicacy will be coyly respected. This is a signal for the patients to take over: "How long have you been mainlining?" "Snorting? Sniffing? Pure cocaine? Man! Three years?" "Busted!" "Listen . . . I could use 80 of meth for hair tonic . . . just doesn't touch me," "I been here twice . . . tried Phoenix, Sera . . ." etc. Soon the relatives are listening in bewilderment, fascination, or horror; they are out and the patients are in, and the therapists are maneuvering to get the session back to where they want it, that is, to some meaningful exchange among family members and within the group.

Vi is slumped down, legs apart and stretched out before her, cigarette held between thumb and forefinger. She squints, shrugs and giggles as her sister loudly says, "Well, we were brought up in the same house and *I* didn't become an addict. . . . I suppose I'm closer to my mother . . . more . . . I just wasn't attracted to it . . . but I have faith she will make it. . . . I know she wants to stop. . . . I have faith in her. . . ." She looks around smugly and defiantly. Vi's mother lifts her shoulders helplessly and says in English and Spanish, "If I had call Brooklyn and tol' your father he wouldda beat the shit outa you."

Mr. A. then explains his long haul through A.A. and his pride in "licking drink," while Jean pats him on the thigh, smiles benignly and says, "If my old man can make it, me too!" They are seductive with one another while they describe their physical quarrels that led to hair-pulling and rolling on the floor.

Jean (becoming angry): G'wan! Every time I gotta welfare check you're on my back.

Father (to Jean): I don't want the money . . . but you can't handle it . . . just trying to stop you. . . .

Ray (to Jean): You got a father, why don' ya pleez 'im?

Pat (interrupting): All I want is to get my kid back . . . that's why I'm here. . . . I'll go back to my methadone counselor. . . .

Therapist (to Pat): But you were drinking and you're playing around with your life.

Mrs. L. (to Therapist): I can understand . . . she's anxious . . . maybe a tranquilizer. . . . I don't know how I can help her. When she's home

. . . I've got arthritis, I can't work anymore. She should help. She just sits around.

Pat (to Mrs. L.): I've got a kid of my own and you treat me like one! I just want to get out and have my own place. . . .

Mrs. L.: You can't make it on your own. How can. . . .

Ray (to Mrs. L.): She's gotta make it on her own.

Vi (to Ray): She and the mother got each other. They could live together and Pat shoulda helped her.

(Vi's mother snorts and looks around restlessly.)

Ray (to no one in particular): The only time I feel like myself was when I shot up . . . it wasn't my sister or my mother . . . man, it was *me!*

The lack of generation boundaries, the loose concepts of time, personal space and age-appropriate behavior, the use or abuse of one another for money, and the jockeying for position within the family while attempting to "differentiate" are revealed. Other examples of this are apparent in the following:

> "He should go to jail? Never! My son? He is not a bum!"
> "Joe, be a man. Have willpower . . . come to work on the truck with me and soon you'll own the business!"
> "Pop, I could buy you twice over with the money I've handled with junk!" (Father smiles with pride.)

The chaotic existence is reproduced in the group by disjunctive communication, and the lack of responsiveness to other families, to spouse or children. Disjunctive communication was also evidenced when people spoke out into the middle space and not to any one in particular. Interruptions were frequent and were used to obfuscate a message, not to assert a position or clarify an idea. This was particularly evident when a parent or spouse "took over" for the patient, or excitement was generated through a simple or deliberate misunderstanding and capitalized on to create further exchange, or contact.

The chaos in the family living was also apparent in the looseness and vagueness of information given in reply to such questions as who lives with whom, when, or why. This seemed partly due to the transiency of the addict's life on the street; for many it was a means of solving behavioral or economic problems by *removal* of child, spouse or oneself.

We have recognized certain family "roles" in these sessions. One is that of "pusher" in the family, usually the member who has the greatest vested interest in contributing to and perpetrating the addiction. This could be a parent who found it possible to use the addict's problems to gratify his/her own unmet needs, or a sibling who found she could take advantage of being the "good one," or very commonly a spouse or lover who was the "easy rider" (Wellisch, 1970) and directly exploitive. The "pusher" could be a parent, aunt, or grandparent who was competing with the other family members to be considered the "understanding one." An example of this, somewhat extreme, but basically characteristic, is a parent who claimed he was helping his 14-year-old addicted son by going through the experience with him. "I did everything but shoot up with him. I was getting into his mind, see, so I could understand him and get him out of drugs." In the process the boy was inducting the father to the street life: where to buy heroin, how to buy it and its effects. Another example of a "pusher" in the family is the spouse who, listening as her husband prepares his "works," knows she won't be "hassled about sex" and says, "when he is on drugs, we don't fight . . . much easier to get along." Another is the "respectable" woman benefiting materially from the money her husband gets from pushing in order to maintain his own habit, although she says she is strongly against drugs!

We look for the designated role of the addict member. In addition to the obvious scapegoat role, there are the less apparent roles of interpreter within the family, go-between, and the *supplier*. The later applies to one who has attempted to pull the family together by trying to be whatever other family members need him or her to be (a substitute spouse, lover, brother, or friend). An example is four young men whose role in their families was to attend to the needs of "sickly" mothers as well as help the fathers. The fathers were harassed men striving to establish their own small businesses. These boys had been chosen to supply the affectional deprivation of both parents. The confusion of these alliances may have contributed to the ease with which these boys prostituted for drugs, while they lived with their girl friends.

We try to identify the characteristic means the addict member had developed for "turning-on" the other family members, that is, the nature of his/her power over the others in the family—the power to manipulate the feelings of the family by being "sick," by creating crises, by rallying the family resources to keep him alive or out of jail. Since we know that to have such power requires some kind of tacit agreement with at least two other family members, we attempt to identify these particular alliances. (We believe that this question of the "power" of the addict vis-à-vis the family requires deeper explorations.) We do suggest that it is utilized by the family to feed an illusion of closeness. By his activities the addicted adolescent functions as an ineffective glue for the family.

The second stage of the MFT is characterized by the therapists' confrontations with what has been observed of the interactions, the family structure and "dynamics." These elicit denials, accusations of not understanding, etc., and can result in a family cohesion vis-à-vis the therapists. The group may support the family or the therapists depending on how similar the other families' situations are to the one being addressed. The therapists' efforts are directed at exposing conscious or unconscious support of the addict by some family members.

Excerpts from a Third Session

Although this session was attended by other families the exchanges here are primarily within the B. family—Debby the patient, age 19, Mr. B., a post office employee, and Mrs. B., a domestic worker, both in their late 40's, and three other children, boys, whose ages range from 14 to 17. This is an intact family, except that Mr. B. does not always sleep at home, and Mrs. B. suspects he has another woman. Mrs. B.'s strong religious beliefs are expressed in her statement, "Debby's future is in God's hands." Mrs. B. feels she can do no more. Debby has obvious homosexual characteristics. Her mother indirectly referred to this in a previous session by complaining that it "isn't natural" for a girl not to have dates. Debby's addiction had caused one crisis after another (running to hospitals, pulling her off the street—each son at one time or another had been sent to look for her).

The brothers were very quiet and embarrassed during the session. While disengaging themselves from Debby, they let it be known that they knew "the street," and knew Debby's connections and the fact that she hustled. They were willing to help, but it was apparent that they resented Debby and her alliance with their father. A discussion had just occurred in which Mrs. B. had complained that Mr. B. did not act like "a man" around the house, that he didn't take care of things. Mr. B. said it was time the boys took over. He was tired, and old; he shouldn't have to bother; "I broke my back all my life and still have nothing." Mrs. B. complained of his drinking, his favoring Debby, and his lack of understanding about the boys. The therapists were pointing out the split in the family.

Therapist (to Mr. B.): You know you have given her carfare before and she used it for drugs, and she took money from her mother's purse.

She pawned the radio and you still give her money. Your wife doesn't like that and. . . .

Mr. B. (defiantly): It's better for Debby to steal from the family than other people. When she takes it from her brothers I pay it back to them. Sometimes she doesn't even know.

Mrs. B. (interrupting, looking at Debby): She always got around him. She twists him around. She comes in high . . . when I give her food she dumps it all over . . . messes up.

Mr. B. (interrupting, to Therapist): The money's for the carfare. She's supposed to get welfare while she's on a program. That's the trouble! Why they give that to her? It's all she waitin' for.

Debby (to mother, resignedly): Chris'! I'm signin' outta here. I'm always in the middle.

Mr. B. (angrily, to Therapist): This not doin' good. She better off at home. . . .

Mrs. B. (to Therapist): What we gonna do?

Therapist: You're all doing your thing. . . .

Mr. B. (to Mrs. B.): I say she can go home! Don' I pay the bills?

Debby (to Mrs. B.): I'll get my own place soon. I can make it on my own . . . this time . . . do it cold.

Therapist: You said you're going to a program.

Debby: I can do it on my own. I'm no goddam baby . . . am I?

Mr. and Mrs. B. agree to let Debby come home "if she promises to stay away from drugs." *This is the fourth hospitalization for Debby.* The therapists expose the interactions: Mr. B.'s protection of Debby; his allowing his disagreements with his wife to ensnare Debby again; Mrs. B.'s apparent helplessness; Debby's collusion with her father even though she complains of "being in the middle"; her challenging the parents' tolerance; their response by accepting her home again for their own needs. Her claim "I'm no baby" is half assertion, half question. The therapists point out how she has relinquished her own plans. The group participates by urging Debby to reconsider and to enter a drug-free resident program.

The last stage ideally culminates in a decision and a plan. The decision-making process (drug-free treatment, methadone maintenance, self-help and home, or back to the street) is fraught with tensions and conflicts. The struggles are related to assertions of parental authority over the adolescent's preferences and the addict's power to maintain anxiety in the others.

In one-third of the cases the plans remain nebulous. This seems at times to be due to the fact that the addict is unconvinced of his family's real support, or to his own unwillingness to accept the discipline of a treatment center. When the addict member announces his decision to the group the reactions waver between supportive comments and sadness when his indecision is obvious.

The family members express fear and resentment of the transition. The addict talks of what it is like to walk out and "meet the street," of the challenges, frustrations and temptations. Parents of the younger adolescents express their fear of the old friends, *or of the separation.* The therapists emphasize that the parents have the capacity to exert control in their own home, and that change is possible.

The therapists are usually left with the feeling of unfinished business, of having gained knowledge that could be helpful if given the opportunity to work longer with some of the families. The limitations of four or six sessions are particularly onerous when an addict's ambiguity about his plans indicates his decision to continue on drugs.

Addicted Couples Groups

The couples groups follow similar patterns but the content is somewhat different. The major themes of this group are sexual problems, demoralizing activity of one partner or the other when either decides to stop drugs, and resentments towards a partner's parents for placing blame on the spouse for drug abuse. Isolation and loneliness are given as reasons for remaining together and, frequently, helplessness in the care of children.

These couples, even more than the parent and adolescent groups, gave cliché responses explaining their relationships: "We love one another," "we couldn't stay apart," "love at first sight," etc. When confronted with the real nature of their relationships they seemed incapable of recognizing the contradiction between parasitism and lovingness. They felt it was better to be together than to be alone, even though there were the abuses generated by hostility and contempt for one another. An example of this is the young man who talks of his "heavy" feeling when his "wife" prostitutes for their money, but believes she is "too stupid to get around alone . . . needs a strong man, and besides, she knows what I'm like. . . . I know her." Or, "He took the welfare money . . . left me without a cent, so, I took the kids to his mother, but we always get back together."

Another significant element in the relationship was the belief or fantasy that this partner was or could be so perceptive that "ordinary" ways of communicating could be transcended. "He knows what I mean" or, "She really understands. I don't have to say it. We just have to look . . . and we know."

The sexual difficulties the couples report are a result of growing indifference to sex, the male's concomitant aggressive stance of masculinity, and on the girl's part, a superior, but secretly relieved, attitude. Both men and women showed extraordinary confusions, misinformation and ignorances about sexual functionings. (A number of young men believed that girls were capable of having orgasms by simply crossing their legs, and were doing so all the time.) They generally agreed that sex was better when they were both "high," however, more of the women tried to articulate dissatisfaction with the absence of a sense of intimacy or personalness during sex.

Three sources of quarrels were common: conflict over money, whether to spend it on drugs or home needs; attempts of a partner to pull the other away from the family of origin; and perhaps the most irritating, the *covert* expectations of the man for an efficient homemaker and of the woman for a good provider. It seemed that each spouse hoped the partner and the marital alliance would be the *vehicle* for attaining the benefits and advantages of a "straight life," without any individual struggle. Since the couples engaged in the actual practice of abuse and derogation of one another while maintaining unrealistic expectations, the arguments were rarely resolved except through more drugs or separations.

Many of the women of these couples were pregnant at the time. Discussion in the group revealed that the young man's fascination with being a father was so romanticized that "planning" for a baby went no further than a week or two hence. We found that in more than half of the couples (35) seen in these groups the young man pressured for the birth of a child and the partner usually acknowledged she was "doing it for him." Reasons given were that this seemed the only way to keep her partner, but if he still left her, then she would have the child to love her. However, when some of these women went to resident treatment they later expressed great anger and bitterness with the partner, recognizing that they had been used, but with little awareness of how they themselves made it possible.

The role-structures that were being developed by these couples (those that had been together at least a year) were extremes, almost caricatures, of the traditional, conventional nuclear family. This was a source of much of the anger and violence between the partners, the need to be "given" the attributes of a home, household, and marriage. For the man it meant to be *viewed* as the protector of the girl, and to be able to view "his woman" as needy, ineffectual, but loving. However, the girl generally gave lip service support to this concept of marriage; she maintained a conviction of her ability and necessity to manipulate as the "power behind the throne," while anxiously and privately preparing herself for the dissolution of the relationship.

Decision-making for these young people as couples was turbulent. The therapeutic intervention here was to help each partner discuss what plan was best for him or her and then urge discussion of what it meant for them as a couple. In some instances partners separated as a result of being in the group. Efforts to direct each to a resident program or even day-care could be defeated by a partner's inability to accept separation; however, suggested plans that might strengthen a "marital-contract," i.e. a methadone clinic providing couples' counseling, were resisted with arguments in favor of a drug-free program. This resistance reflected not only uncertainty in relinquishing drugs and the attendant life-style, but was intertwined with the desire to keep the "marital contract" loose and flexible. In some instances it meant maintaining the prerogatives of exploitation. Their purposes in attending the group (even after discharge from detoxification) seemed to be in the hope of transforming the therapist's concern into a motivation for a new life. They reflected, in the group, the process described by Mead and Campbell (1972)—the absence of spontaneous agreement or self-revealing reasons for disagreement. They tended to use open and veiled threats to coerce and maintain the status quo.

The explorations of the nature of the relationship were threatening to the myths of closeness and intimacy and often broke into the illusions of the partner or expected child as "savior." Also, the power of the need to experience or be experienced as "two against the world" was frequently stronger than the impact of the group and therapists.

The addicted couples present a challenging problem in treatment and counseling. These very young adult and adolescent marital alliances, bonded by a common addiction and determined by the necessary life-style, seem to produce a condensation and compression of all the complexities, miseries and discords in the formation of a modern "nuclear family." *They develop with a rapid velocity*. An incident that illustrates this is the insistence of a patient that he be allowed into the couples group because his wife had died recently from an overdose of heroin which he had hustled and given to her. He "wanted to be with other couples and mourn her" and to talk about his two-year-old child who was with his mother. He was 23, but he looked and talked like an old man. His expectation and desire for a quick relief from anxiety were palpable; more to the point was his sensation that he and his wife had been through the whole life cycle together.

Parent-Couples Group

The following is a report on a parent-couples group whose children were in a resident program. Some of these families had attended the short-term MFT in the detoxification program. This group was an initial experiment in a situation where *extracting the addict from the total environment* was considered necessary.

After more than a year or even two years of stay in resident treatment, the adolescent faces reentry to the family. Unless both adolescent and parents are prepared for the reentry the ex-addict can be pulled into former family roles by the suction of the family "system." The family can be disrupted in its current organization by the returning member. We considered this situation as contributing to recidivism.

(The following was reported by Pauline Kaufman, clinical consultant to Phoenix Program.) As an experiment in prevention, one Phoenix house, a therapeutic community in New York City, invited seven parent-couples to visit with a family therapist, once a week for six months. The criteria for selection for this initial effort were that both parents, patient and children be living together, that the patient be 17 or under, that some of the siblings be close to the age of the addict, and that the families be representative of the ethnic and class background of the residents. (These class groups were the same as described for the detoxification groups.) The goals of these sessions were similar to those stated for groups already described, except for certain differences. The therapists were working in a milieu created by the commitment to change, past the point of decision, and they had knowledge of the patients for an extended time span. Therefore, their focus was on working through some of the pathologically rigidified interactions within the family.

This group consisted of two Puerto Rican parent-couples, two black, and three white—Irish, Italian and Jewish. All were low-income families; all had been on welfare a number of times, and lived in ghetto areas. The siblings ranged from 4 to 18 years old. The fathers were all in unskilled or semiskilled trades and the mothers had worked sporadically.

All of these parents were born in this country. The parents' ages were from 28 to 55; the ages of the seven patients were 13 (a boy and a girl), 14 (two boys), 15 (a boy and a girl), and 17 (one boy). Completing the group was a white therapist, three trainees who were former addicts—two blacks, and one Puerto Rican.

The initial phases for this group were determined by the therapists' emphasis on the fact that the children were 17 or under and probably would be returning home.

The atmosphere of the group was, at the beginning, characterized by excitement, intensity and rapid discharges of tension occurring through sudden spurts of talk eagerly directed towards the staff. The noise level was high as the expressions of anxiety and fear emerged. The major themes were fear of a return to addiction, fear of "contagion" of the other children, and feelings of helplessness in dealing with the returning children.

These fears were elaborated on in the ensuing sessions. Other problems within the family emerged as we considered these apprehensions. By the sixth session the members had developed an understanding of the addicted child as a "symptom-bearer" of the family troubles. Here there existed an opportunity to pin down and work more intensively with a family member who was giving implicit or tacit permission for drug use.

Before change could be effected a period of time was required for the ventilation of anger and resentment. Within this time the terrible "neediness" of these families became flagrantly apparent. The common expressions of it were such statements as:

"He/she has disregarded *us*."
"We are poor people; we have no time."
"We need more help than he does. We're tired."
"She has had it good here . . . meals, sleep . . . let her learn to make her own way."
"We are sick . . . both of us."
"He owes *us* something."
"She should of helped us. . . ."

By the 12th session parental discord could be aired in the group, and negotiations for resolutions of some conflicts could occur, as illustrated by the following:

Ray, the teenage son, had been in the program for almost a year. His counselor had discussed with him the possibility of a visit home for the weekend. The group discussed the fact that Mrs. M. had not told her husband. She explained, "He is tired. It isn't necessary to worry him about Ray." Mr. M. was angry; he asserted he is the father and should be told such things; he accused her of being frightened of him and protective of Ray, or of babying him. He claimed it is her fault that Ray expects too much; she should pay more attention to the home and the other children.

The exchange between them elicited expressions of anxiety and criticism from other participants. Mrs. J. said "I'm ill. I have to go to the hospital soon." Others suggested the M.s aren't ready to have Ray home, and Ray's counselor reported that Ray is scared of the visit. As the session moved on the altercation between the M.s revolved around where Ray would sleep. (His bed had been in the parents' bedroom.) There had been an attempt to keep the livingroom free of beds. Mr. M. insisted that Ray sleep on the couch. Mrs. M. claimed Ray would not like that and it would lead to trouble. She appeared subtly threatening in her manner. A member pointed out that they should either get together about things before Ray's visit or cancel it. The M.s asserted they both wanted Ray home. Mrs. M. agreed that Ray should sleep on the couch, if Mr. M. agreed not to get riled up and to yell and shout, but rather to *talk* to Ray and, maybe, to try to do something special with him. The therapist suggested that they could help each other if something occurred that scared them and pointed out that they had learned to talk to one another and control anger enough to be able to negotiate.

This family interaction demonstrated some confusion of roles that had developed in the M. family and the efforts made to clarify them. This excerpt is lifted out of a session in which there was much more going on than can be reported. It does, however, show the beginnings of an opening up for the M. family when faced with Ray's reentry.

Prior to this session the M.s had closed ranks and this had given the family a semblance of healthy functioning. Worry and talk about Ray were tolerable as long as he remained outside. Closing the family circle defended against further pain, shame and intrusion, particularly since the other children were not in trouble, but were vulnerable. The conflicts around Ray had gone underground, and in this interim period (not quite a year) there had been a tentative restructuring of parents and children, literally and figuratively. Mrs. M. revealed the tentativeness by her renewed effort to position Ray between herself and her husband.

Ray's advocate, staff member A., strove to reinforce Ray's right to be a child. And Mr. M. struggled to sustain his position as husband and father. As these struggles became more explicit the anxiety in the group increased, expressed by Mrs. J.'s reference to illness, and by staff member A.'s need to refocus on Ray and avoid a response to Mrs. J. Mrs. M.'s need for Ray as a closet supporter and her indulgences of him in the past, perhaps as payment, were exposed and are less likely to recur.

In the weeks following, almost all the couples demonstrated similar fears and struggles for and against the former roles and alliances, as the adolescents' return became a reality. Each family's experience was shared and worked with, in the group. As the group developed a pool of common experiences, problems were solved more rapidly.

Communication, which in the beginning was limited to expression of anger, frustration and pain, began to be used as a way of getting and giving information and of giving and getting support. The members showed greater tolerance for another person's pain, and became less inclined to offer quick solutions. After three months they spoke of providing routines in family life, of finding alternatives to just "letting it all hang out," and reported that "rapping" became a family pattern.

The relationships between the parent-couples showed greater tenderness. The view of the spouse as adversary decreased as they tended to look outward for the enemy rather than inward to one another. Further, they were less likely to convert the frustrations of their poverty into quarrels that had, in the past, injured the partner's self-esteem.

After the adolescent returned and lived and functioned together with the family it was common when a crisis occurred for the *whole family* to return for a session; they did not fall back on scapegoating and dumping all the family problems on the addiction. The family members could perceive problems more discretely. None of the siblings close in age to the addicted members became addicted to drugs or alcohol, and five of the patients had remained totally drug-free a year after termination. We consider this an important index of growth in the family.

CONCLUSIONS

The MFT groups described illuminate the fact that this modality is helpful in reversing a trend when the patient and the family are both in a crisis and at a point of decision. The group therapies reported represent a minimum of what is required. They are efforts to meet, in a pragmatic way, the necessities of limited time and funds.

The limitations are surely apparent. We found that four to six sessions during detoxification were too often insufficient for transition from the hospital. The need for continuity of family therapies through transitional periods is patently obvious, and when it is absent there is frustration for all.

The limitations of the parent-couples group are due, in part, to its being adjunctive and not integrated to the adolsecents' resident program. Particular difficulties arose around the complex problems related to imminent separation and independence of the adolescent from the family; working for a smooth reentry was often insufficient.

In both situations (detoxification and resident) calls for help derived from the difficulties of attempts to exit from the family. Although family members had learned better ways of interacting with one another at home, troubles developed around the more common and ordinary strains of adolescent self-assertion and the need to break away. The fears of "making it in a straight world" and the parental negations of independence compounded the difficulties of moving on.

The addicted couples group presents the special problems indicated above. The challenges of working with this group do require further investigation; the intensity of their bitterness towards the spouse's family of origin and the evolving ideology of two against the world, as well as the sexual difficulties and rapid role rigidification, all warrant attention.

We do not assume that family therapies described above are by themselves the answers to the problems of adolescents and/or drug addiction. We do believe they are basically helpful in ameliorating some of the stresses in the lives of the families with an addicted member. We are convinced that family therapies should be introduced at the earliest possible moment and considered essential rather than ancillary to the treatment of an addicted adolescent.

What confounds us is what to do when an addict and his family find that society's flirtation with providing job opportunities is a farce, that he or she has learned an unnecessary skill, or that they suffer greater economic stress because welfare is no longer available for an ex-addict. We are also struggling with the problems encountered when our own efforts and anxieties increase as funds for such work decrease. The social milieu is no mere background to the flowering of cynicism in adolescence.

The age of anxiety of 20 and 30 years ago has metamorphosed into the age of cynicism. Drug addiction in youth is a partial expression of both. Anxiety and cynicism are abortive to processes of growth. Thus it is no wonder that the young reflect in their pursuits the avoidance and denial of processes and in turn are enveloped in another unmanageable process.

"There ain't nothing to look at, no place to go—it's just the same in as it is out—might as well go 'up.' "

—*A 14-year-old ghetto boy*

REFERENCES

AUERSWALD, E. (1964). Some clinical observations on the role of cognitive deficits in the development of maladaptive ego states. Presented at American Psychiatric Association, December.

AUERSWALD, E. (1966). Cognitive development and psychopathology. Presented at 5th Annual Conference on Urban Education, Yeshiva University, New York.

FRAMO, J. (1970). Symptoms from a family transactional viewpoint. In *Family Therapy in Transition*. N. Ackerman, ed., pp. 125-171. Boston: Little, Brown.

LAQUEUR, H. P. (1964). Multiple family therapy: Further developments. *International Journal of Social Psychiatry*, Congress Issue, Section R.

LAQUEUR, H. P., ZUNITSH, M. S., SMITH, G. E., and WELLS, C. F. (1969). Multiple family therapy and the decision making process. Presented at 2nd International Congress of Social Psychiatry, London.

LAQUEUR, H. P. (1972). Mechanisms of change in multiple family therapy. In *Progress in Group and Family Therapy*, C. Sager and H. S. Kaplan, eds., pp. 400-415. New York: Brunner/Mazel.

MEAD, E., and CAMPBELL, S. (1972). Decision-making and interaction with and without a drug abusing child. *Family Process*, 11:487-498.

MINUCHIN, S. M., MONTALVO, B., GUERNEY, B., ROSMAN, B., and SCHUMER, F. (1967). The disorganized and disadvantaged family. In *Families of the Slums*, pp. 221-229. New York: Basic Books.

WELLISCH, D. (1970). The easy rider syndrome: A pattern of hetero- and homosexual relationships in a heroin addict population. *Family Process*, 9:425-430.

Index

283